# This Health Information Planner belongs to

_____

A cheerful heart is good medicine,
but a broken spirit saps a person's strength.
Holy Bible, Proverbs 17:22 NLT

My Lord, increase me in knowledge.
Taha Qur'an 20:114

PGF Publications
My Health Information Planner
Copyright © 2022 by John and Monette Mottenon

Printed in the United States of America

First Printing, 2022

ISBN: 978-1-955063-60-9

PGF Publications
Montgomery, Alabama

Photo Credit: Mr. Gil Beavers

# My Health Information Planner

A cheerful heart is good medicine, but a broken spirit saps a person's strength.
Holy Bible, Proverbs 17:22 NLT

My Lord, increase me in knowledge.
Taha Qur'an 20:114

# PGF Publications

Holy Bible, Psalm 96:3 – 4 NLT
Publish his glorious deeds among the nations. Tell everyone about the amazing things he does.
Great is the Lord! He is most worthy of praise!

# Notes and Reflections

# MY HEALTH INFORMATION PLANNER
## Table of Contents

**How to Use and Set Up Your**
**"MY HEALTH INFORMATION PLANNER"**     **9**

**Section 1 My General Profile**     **11**

❖ My General Information     **12**

❖ Emergency Contacts     **13**

❖ My Family Information     **15**

❖ My Wellness Tracker     **16**

❖ My Favorites/Preferences     **41**

❖ Family Support Resources     **43**

     o Support Group

     o Religious Group

     o Counseling Service

     o Other Organizations

**Section 2 Calendars**     **45**

❖ Current Yearly Calendar     **46**

❖ Quarterly Calendars     **47**

❖ Next Year Calendar     **51**

**Section 3 Doctor Visits & Question Logs**     **57**

    ❖ Appointment & Question Logs     **58**

    ❖ Doctor/Provider Visit Notes (24)     **63**

    ❖ Equipment Lists     **111**

    ❖ Supplies List     **115**

**Section 4 Health History**     **119**

    ❖ My Health History

    ❖ My Family Health History     **120**

    ❖ Surgeries, Procedures, Vaccinations     **125**

    ❖ Emergency Calls     **127**

    ❖ Hospital Admission Tracking (*Other than surgery*)     **129**

    ❖ My Test Results Log (*include records of blood or urine tests, X-rays, etc.*)     **131**

    ❖ Medical Records from Doctors

**Section 5 Medication Management**     **135**

    ❖ Provider Medication Log     **136**

    ❖ Detailed Medication Management Logs     **139**

    ❖ Diet & Nutrition Notes     **147**

**Section 6 Insurance Information**     **149**

    ❖ Insurance information     **150**

    ❖ Record of Medical Expenses     **153**

## Section 7 Doctor & Business Contacts                          155

❖ Primary Care Providers Contact Information                     157
❖ Specialist Providers Contact Information

❖ General Providers Contact Information

*May include some or all of the following:*

- *Exercise/Recreation Center*
- *Dental Care Provider*
- *Home Health Care Provider*
- *Insurance Case Manager*
- *Durable Medical Equipment Provider*

- *Medicaid*
- *Transportation*
- *Social Services*
- *Respite Care*

- *Therapists*
- *Elder Care*
- *Hospice Services*
- *Clinic Coordinator*

❖ Business Card pages                                            162

## Section 8 Miscellaneous Documents                            165
*(Insert copies of correspondence including appointment letters, insurance referral authorization letter, etc.)*

## About the Authors                                            167

# Notes and Reflections

_____
_____
_____
_____
_____
_____
_____
_____
_____
_____
_____
_____
_____
_____
_____
_____
_____
_____
_____
_____
_____
_____
_____
_____
_____

## HOW TO USE YOUR "MY HEALTH INFORMATION PLANNER"

It is more important than ever to keep track of your health care records. It can be overwhelming to visit your health care provider and remember all of your health history as well as your family's health history. This "MY HEALTH INFORMATION PLANNER" is designed to help you maintain a continuous record of your care, services, providers, notes, documents, and more.

Health professionals will appreciate you bringing your "MY HEALTH INFORMATION PLANNER" to each medical appointment, therapy, on vacations, etc. This will ensure that information is kept updated and available in the time of need. Work with your health professionals as a team by asking for copies of visit notes, immunization records, medical records, doctor reports, and other information. Insert this information into your "MY HEALTH INFORMATION PLANNER" for safe keeping.

## HOW DO I SET UP "MY HEALTH INFORMATION PLANNER"

1. MY HEALTH INFORMATION PLANNERS are very personal to you and should be customized to reflect your medical history and current information. Use pages that are most important to you. It may seem overwhelming to complete, but once the information is complete, you'll just need to keep it updated after each appointment or at least once per month.

2. Gather your information that you already have concerning your health. This may include reports from recent doctor's visits, a recent summary of a hospital stay, names and phone numbers of physicians, hospitals, and relatives. It may also include test results. Business cards can be stored at the back of Section 7.

3. File the information you want to keep in the appropriate section as it is received.

4. *UPDATE* your "MY HEALTH INFORMATION PLANNER" after each visit. To order additional copies of "MY HEALTH INFORMATION PLANNER" contact (334) 219-9300 or visit PGFEducation.com.

5. *ADD* information to your "MY HEALTH INFORMATION PLANNER" as it becomes available. Remember to update medication logs and test logs, etc. Track expenses including store receipts, bills, etc. in an envelope that can be inserted in your "My Health Information Planner." This is great for tax purposes. Enjoy the convenience of having all of your health information handy!

# Notes and Reflections

_____
_____
_____
_____
_____
_____
_____
_____
_____
_____
_____
_____
_____
_____
_____
_____
_____
_____
_____
_____
_____
_____
_____

# Section 1
# My General Profile

- ❖ **My General Information**
- ❖ **Emergency Contacts**
- ❖ **My Family Information**
- ❖ **My Favorites/Preferences**
- ❖ **My Wellness Tracker**
- ❖ **Family Support Resources**
  - o **Support Group**
  - o **Religious Group**
  - o **Counseling Service**
  - o **Other Organizations**

# MY GENERAL INFORMATION

Cover Space with
my current picture

My name is _____ My nickname is _____

My birthday is _____/_____/_____ Height _____ Weight_____

| My Emergency Contacts | | |
|---|---|---|
| Name | Relationship | Contact phone number with area code |
| | | |
| | | |
| | | |
| | | |
| | | |
| | | |
| | | |
| | | |
| | | |

# If you have a separate sheet, of Emergency Contacts, glue them on this page. If not, you can ignore this page.

# Notes and Reflections

# MY FAMILY INFORMATION

My Name _____ My Nickname _____

My Date of Birth _____ My Social Security # _____

Language Spoken at home _____ Interpreter needed Yes ☐     No ☐

Preferred Interpreter _____

Blood Type _____ Ever had a transfusion Yes ☐  No ☐

Primary Diagnosis _____

Secondary Diagnosis _____

Additional Diagnoses _____

_____

_____

_____

My Address _____

City _____ State _____ Zip Code _____

Email Address _____

Phone # Home _____ Mobile _____

Spouse's Name _____

Address _____

City _____ State _____ Zip Code _____

Email Address _____

Phone # Home _____ Mobile _____

# Notes and Reflections

_____

_____

_____

_____

_____

_____

_____

_____

_____

_____

_____

_____

_____

_____

_____

_____

_____

_____

_____

_____

_____

_____

**My Wellness Tracker**

Month of _____

3 Month Goal _____

Goal for the Month _____

Tiny Step for the Week 1 _____

|  | M | T | W | T | F | S | S | Notes |
|---|---|---|---|---|---|---|---|---|
| Steps | | | | | | | | |
| Workout | | | | | | | | |
| Water | | | | | | | | |
| Blood Pressure | | | | | | | | |
| Weight/Pulse | | | | | | | | |

Tiny Step for the Week 2 _____

|  | M | T | W | T | F | S | S | Notes |
|---|---|---|---|---|---|---|---|---|
| Steps | | | | | | | | |
| Workout | | | | | | | | |
| Water | | | | | | | | |
| Blood Pressure | | | | | | | | |
| Weight/Pulse | | | | | | | | |

Tiny Step for the Week 3 _____

|  | M | T | W | T | F | S | S | Notes |
|---|---|---|---|---|---|---|---|---|
| Steps | | | | | | | | |
| Workout | | | | | | | | |
| Water | | | | | | | | |
| Blood Pressure | | | | | | | | |
| Weight/Pulse | | | | | | | | |

Tiny Step for the Week 4 _____

|  | M | T | W | T | F | S | S | Notes |
|---|---|---|---|---|---|---|---|---|
| Steps | | | | | | | | |
| Workout | | | | | | | | |
| Water | | | | | | | | |
| Blood Pressure | | | | | | | | |
| Weight/Pulse | | | | | | | | |

**Monthly Measurements**

|  | Current | Change |  | Current | Change |  | Current | Change |
|---|---|---|---|---|---|---|---|---|
| Bust | | | Hips | | | BMI | | |
| Waist | | | Thigh | | | BF | | |
| Abdomen | | | Arm | | | Other | | |

# Notes and Reflections

_____
_____
_____
_____
_____
_____
_____
_____
_____
_____
_____
_____
_____
_____
_____
_____
_____
_____
_____
_____
_____
_____

# My Wellness Tracker

Month of _____

3 Month Goal _____

Goal for the Month _____

Tiny Step for the Week 1 _____

|  | M | T | W | T | F | S | S | Notes |
|---|---|---|---|---|---|---|---|---|
| Steps |  |  |  |  |  |  |  |  |
| Workout |  |  |  |  |  |  |  |  |
| Water |  |  |  |  |  |  |  |  |
| Blood Pressure |  |  |  |  |  |  |  |  |
| Weight/Pulse |  |  |  |  |  |  |  |  |

Tiny Step for the Week 2 _____

|  | M | T | W | T | F | S | S | Notes |
|---|---|---|---|---|---|---|---|---|
| Steps |  |  |  |  |  |  |  |  |
| Workout |  |  |  |  |  |  |  |  |
| Water |  |  |  |  |  |  |  |  |
| Blood Pressure |  |  |  |  |  |  |  |  |
| Weight/Pulse |  |  |  |  |  |  |  |  |

Tiny Step for the Week 3 _____

|  | M | T | W | T | F | S | S | Notes |
|---|---|---|---|---|---|---|---|---|
| Steps |  |  |  |  |  |  |  |  |
| Workout |  |  |  |  |  |  |  |  |
| Water |  |  |  |  |  |  |  |  |
| Blood Pressure |  |  |  |  |  |  |  |  |
| Weight/Pulse |  |  |  |  |  |  |  |  |

Tiny Step for the Week 4 _____

|  | M | T | W | T | F | S | S | Notes |
|---|---|---|---|---|---|---|---|---|
| Steps |  |  |  |  |  |  |  |  |
| Workout |  |  |  |  |  |  |  |  |
| Water |  |  |  |  |  |  |  |  |
| Blood Pressure |  |  |  |  |  |  |  |  |
| Weight/Pulse |  |  |  |  |  |  |  |  |

## Monthly Measurements

|  | Current | Change |  | Current | Change |  | Current | Change |
|---|---|---|---|---|---|---|---|---|
| Bust |  |  | Hips |  |  | BMI |  |  |
| Waist |  |  | Thigh |  |  | BF |  |  |
| Abdomen |  |  | Arm |  |  | Other |  |  |

# Notes and Reflections

# My Wellness Tracker

Month of _____

3 Month Goal _____

Goal for the Month _____

Tiny Step for the Week 1 _____

|  | M | T | W | T | F | S | S | Notes |
|---|---|---|---|---|---|---|---|---|
| Steps | | | | | | | | |
| Workout | | | | | | | | |
| Water | | | | | | | | |
| Blood Pressure | | | | | | | | |
| Weight/Pulse | | | | | | | | |

Tiny Step for the Week 2 _____

|  | M | T | W | T | F | S | S | Notes |
|---|---|---|---|---|---|---|---|---|
| Steps | | | | | | | | |
| Workout | | | | | | | | |
| Water | | | | | | | | |
| Blood Pressure | | | | | | | | |
| Weight/Pulse | | | | | | | | |

Tiny Step for the Week 3 _____

|  | M | T | W | T | F | S | S | Notes |
|---|---|---|---|---|---|---|---|---|
| Steps | | | | | | | | |
| Workout | | | | | | | | |
| Water | | | | | | | | |
| Blood Pressure | | | | | | | | |
| Weight/Pulse | | | | | | | | |

Tiny Step for the Week 4 _____

|  | M | T | W | T | F | S | S | Notes |
|---|---|---|---|---|---|---|---|---|
| Steps | | | | | | | | |
| Workout | | | | | | | | |
| Water | | | | | | | | |
| Blood Pressure | | | | | | | | |
| Weight/Pulse | | | | | | | | |

## Monthly Measurements

|  | Current | Change |  | Current | Change |  | Current | Change |
|---|---|---|---|---|---|---|---|---|
| Bust | | | Hips | | | BMI | | |
| Waist | | | Thigh | | | BF | | |
| Abdomen | | | Arm | | | Other | | |

# Notes and Reflections

_____
_____
_____
_____
_____
_____
_____
_____
_____
_____
_____
_____
_____
_____
_____
_____
_____
_____
_____
_____
_____
_____
_____

# My Wellness Tracker

Month of _____

3 Month Goal _____

Goal for the Month _____

Tiny Step for the Week 1 _____

|  | M | T | W | T | F | S | S | Notes |
|---|---|---|---|---|---|---|---|---|
| Steps |  |  |  |  |  |  |  |  |
| Workout |  |  |  |  |  |  |  |  |
| Water |  |  |  |  |  |  |  |  |
| Blood Pressure |  |  |  |  |  |  |  |  |
| Weight/Pulse |  |  |  |  |  |  |  |  |

Tiny Step for the Week 2 _____

|  | M | T | W | T | F | S | S | Notes |
|---|---|---|---|---|---|---|---|---|
| Steps |  |  |  |  |  |  |  |  |
| Workout |  |  |  |  |  |  |  |  |
| Water |  |  |  |  |  |  |  |  |
| Blood Pressure |  |  |  |  |  |  |  |  |
| Weight/Pulse |  |  |  |  |  |  |  |  |

Tiny Step for the Week 3 _____

|  | M | T | W | T | F | S | S | Notes |
|---|---|---|---|---|---|---|---|---|
| Steps |  |  |  |  |  |  |  |  |
| Workout |  |  |  |  |  |  |  |  |
| Water |  |  |  |  |  |  |  |  |
| Blood Pressure |  |  |  |  |  |  |  |  |
| Weight/Pulse |  |  |  |  |  |  |  |  |

Tiny Step for the Week 4 _____

|  | M | T | W | T | F | S | S | Notes |
|---|---|---|---|---|---|---|---|---|
| Steps |  |  |  |  |  |  |  |  |
| Workout |  |  |  |  |  |  |  |  |
| Water |  |  |  |  |  |  |  |  |
| Blood Pressure |  |  |  |  |  |  |  |  |
| Weight/Pulse |  |  |  |  |  |  |  |  |

## Monthly Measurements

|  | Current | Change |  | Current | Change |  | Current | Change |
|---|---|---|---|---|---|---|---|---|
| Bust |  |  | Hips |  |  | BMI |  |  |
| Waist |  |  | Thigh |  |  | BF |  |  |
| Abdomen |  |  | Arm |  |  | Other |  |  |

# Notes and Reflections

# My Wellness Tracker

Month of _____

3 Month Goal _____

Goal for the Month _____

Tiny Step for the Week 1 _____

|  | M | T | W | T | F | S | S | Notes |
|---|---|---|---|---|---|---|---|---|
| Steps |  |  |  |  |  |  |  |  |
| Workout |  |  |  |  |  |  |  |  |
| Water |  |  |  |  |  |  |  |  |
| Blood Pressure |  |  |  |  |  |  |  |  |
| Weight/Pulse |  |  |  |  |  |  |  |  |

Tiny Step for the Week 2 _____

|  | M | T | W | T | F | S | S | Notes |
|---|---|---|---|---|---|---|---|---|
| Steps |  |  |  |  |  |  |  |  |
| Workout |  |  |  |  |  |  |  |  |
| Water |  |  |  |  |  |  |  |  |
| Blood Pressure |  |  |  |  |  |  |  |  |
| Weight/Pulse |  |  |  |  |  |  |  |  |

Tiny Step for the Week 3 _____

|  | M | T | W | T | F | S | S | Notes |
|---|---|---|---|---|---|---|---|---|
| Steps |  |  |  |  |  |  |  |  |
| Workout |  |  |  |  |  |  |  |  |
| Water |  |  |  |  |  |  |  |  |
| Blood Pressure |  |  |  |  |  |  |  |  |
| Weight/Pulse |  |  |  |  |  |  |  |  |

Tiny Step for the Week 4 _____

|  | M | T | W | T | F | S | S | Notes |
|---|---|---|---|---|---|---|---|---|
| Steps |  |  |  |  |  |  |  |  |
| Workout |  |  |  |  |  |  |  |  |
| Water |  |  |  |  |  |  |  |  |
| Blood Pressure |  |  |  |  |  |  |  |  |
| Weight/Pulse |  |  |  |  |  |  |  |  |

## Monthly Measurements

|  | Current | Change |  | Current | Change |  | Current | Change |
|---|---|---|---|---|---|---|---|---|
| Bust |  |  | Hips |  |  | BMI |  |  |
| Waist |  |  | Thigh |  |  | BF |  |  |
| Abdomen |  |  | Arm |  |  | Other |  |  |

# Notes and Reflections

# My Wellness Tracker

Month of _____

3 Month Goal _____

Goal for the Month _____

Tiny Step for the Week 1 _____

| | M | T | W | T | F | S | S | Notes |
|---|---|---|---|---|---|---|---|---|
| Steps | | | | | | | | |
| Workout | | | | | | | | |
| Water | | | | | | | | |
| Blood Pressure | | | | | | | | |
| Weight/Pulse | | | | | | | | |

Tiny Step for the Week 2 _____

| | M | T | W | T | F | S | S | Notes |
|---|---|---|---|---|---|---|---|---|
| Steps | | | | | | | | |
| Workout | | | | | | | | |
| Water | | | | | | | | |
| Blood Pressure | | | | | | | | |
| Weight/Pulse | | | | | | | | |

Tiny Step for the Week 3 _____

| | M | T | W | T | F | S | S | Notes |
|---|---|---|---|---|---|---|---|---|
| Steps | | | | | | | | |
| Workout | | | | | | | | |
| Water | | | | | | | | |
| Blood Pressure | | | | | | | | |
| Weight/Pulse | | | | | | | | |

Tiny Step for the Week 4 _____

| | M | T | W | T | F | S | S | Notes |
|---|---|---|---|---|---|---|---|---|
| Steps | | | | | | | | |
| Workout | | | | | | | | |
| Water | | | | | | | | |
| Blood Pressure | | | | | | | | |
| Weight/Pulse | | | | | | | | |

## Monthly Measurements

| | Current | Change | | Current | Change | | Current | Change |
|---|---|---|---|---|---|---|---|---|
| Bust | | | Hips | | | BMI | | |
| Waist | | | Thigh | | | BF | | |
| Abdomen | | | Arm | | | Other | | |

# Notes and Reflections

_____
_____
_____
_____
_____
_____
_____
_____
_____
_____
_____
_____
_____
_____
_____
_____
_____
_____
_____
_____
_____
_____
_____

# My Wellness Tracker

Month of _____

3 Month Goal _____

Goal for the Month _____

Tiny Step for the Week 1 _____

| | M | T | W | T | F | S | S | Notes |
|---|---|---|---|---|---|---|---|---|
| Steps | | | | | | | | |
| Workout | | | | | | | | |
| Water | | | | | | | | |
| Blood Pressure | | | | | | | | |
| Weight/Pulse | | | | | | | | |

Tiny Step for the Week 2 _____

| | M | T | W | T | F | S | S | Notes |
|---|---|---|---|---|---|---|---|---|
| Steps | | | | | | | | |
| Workout | | | | | | | | |
| Water | | | | | | | | |
| Blood Pressure | | | | | | | | |
| Weight/Pulse | | | | | | | | |

Tiny Step for the Week 3 _____

| | M | T | W | T | F | S | S | Notes |
|---|---|---|---|---|---|---|---|---|
| Steps | | | | | | | | |
| Workout | | | | | | | | |
| Water | | | | | | | | |
| Blood Pressure | | | | | | | | |
| Weight/Pulse | | | | | | | | |

Tiny Step for the Week 4 _____

| | M | T | W | T | F | S | S | Notes |
|---|---|---|---|---|---|---|---|---|
| Steps | | | | | | | | |
| Workout | | | | | | | | |
| Water | | | | | | | | |
| Blood Pressure | | | | | | | | |
| Weight/Pulse | | | | | | | | |

## Monthly Measurements

| | Current | Change | | Current | Change | | Current | Change |
|---|---|---|---|---|---|---|---|---|
| Bust | | | Hips | | | BMI | | |
| Waist | | | Thigh | | | BF | | |
| Abdomen | | | Arm | | | Other | | |

# Notes and Reflections

_____
_____
_____
_____
_____
_____
_____
_____
_____
_____
_____
_____
_____
_____
_____
_____
_____
_____
_____
_____
_____
_____
_____

# My Wellness Tracker

Month of _____

3 Month Goal _____

Goal for the Month _____

Tiny Step for the Week 1 _____

|  | M | T | W | T | F | S | S | Notes |
|---|---|---|---|---|---|---|---|---|
| Steps |  |  |  |  |  |  |  |  |
| Workout |  |  |  |  |  |  |  |  |
| Water |  |  |  |  |  |  |  |  |
| Blood Pressure |  |  |  |  |  |  |  |  |
| Weight/Pulse |  |  |  |  |  |  |  |  |

Tiny Step for the Week 2 _____

|  | M | T | W | T | F | S | S | Notes |
|---|---|---|---|---|---|---|---|---|
| Steps |  |  |  |  |  |  |  |  |
| Workout |  |  |  |  |  |  |  |  |
| Water |  |  |  |  |  |  |  |  |
| Blood Pressure |  |  |  |  |  |  |  |  |
| Weight/Pulse |  |  |  |  |  |  |  |  |

Tiny Step for the Week 3 _____

|  | M | T | W | T | F | S | S | Notes |
|---|---|---|---|---|---|---|---|---|
| Steps |  |  |  |  |  |  |  |  |
| Workout |  |  |  |  |  |  |  |  |
| Water |  |  |  |  |  |  |  |  |
| Blood Pressure |  |  |  |  |  |  |  |  |
| Weight/Pulse |  |  |  |  |  |  |  |  |

Tiny Step for the Week 4 _____

|  | M | T | W | T | F | S | S | Notes |
|---|---|---|---|---|---|---|---|---|
| Steps |  |  |  |  |  |  |  |  |
| Workout |  |  |  |  |  |  |  |  |
| Water |  |  |  |  |  |  |  |  |
| Blood Pressure |  |  |  |  |  |  |  |  |
| Weight/Pulse |  |  |  |  |  |  |  |  |

## Monthly Measurements

|  | Current | Change |  | Current | Change |  | Current | Change |
|---|---|---|---|---|---|---|---|---|
| Bust |  |  | Hips |  |  | BMI |  |  |
| Waist |  |  | Thigh |  |  | BF |  |  |
| Abdomen |  |  | Arm |  |  | Other |  |  |

# Notes and Reflections

_____

_____

_____

_____

_____

_____

_____

_____

_____

_____

_____

_____

_____

_____

_____

_____

_____

_____

_____

_____

_____

_____

_____

_____

## My Wellness Tracker

Month of _____

3 Month Goal _____

Goal for the Month _____

Tiny Step for the Week 1 _____

| | M | T | W | T | F | S | S | Notes |
|---|---|---|---|---|---|---|---|---|
| Steps | | | | | | | | |
| Workout | | | | | | | | |
| Water | | | | | | | | |
| Blood Pressure | | | | | | | | |
| Weight/Pulse | | | | | | | | |

Tiny Step for the Week 2 _____

| | M | T | W | T | F | S | S | Notes |
|---|---|---|---|---|---|---|---|---|
| Steps | | | | | | | | |
| Workout | | | | | | | | |
| Water | | | | | | | | |
| Blood Pressure | | | | | | | | |
| Weight/Pulse | | | | | | | | |

Tiny Step for the Week 3 _____

| | M | T | W | T | F | S | S | Notes |
|---|---|---|---|---|---|---|---|---|
| Steps | | | | | | | | |
| Workout | | | | | | | | |
| Water | | | | | | | | |
| Blood Pressure | | | | | | | | |
| Weight/Pulse | | | | | | | | |

Tiny Step for the Week 4 _____

| | M | T | W | T | F | S | S | Notes |
|---|---|---|---|---|---|---|---|---|
| Steps | | | | | | | | |
| Workout | | | | | | | | |
| Water | | | | | | | | |
| Blood Pressure | | | | | | | | |
| Weight/Pulse | | | | | | | | |

### Monthly Measurements

| | Current | Change | | Current | Change | | Current | Change |
|---|---|---|---|---|---|---|---|---|
| Bust | | | Hips | | | BMI | | |
| Waist | | | Thigh | | | BF | | |
| Abdomen | | | Arm | | | Other | | |

# Notes and Reflections

## My Wellness Tracker

Month of _____

3 Month Goal _____

Goal for the Month _____

Tiny Step for the Week 1 _____

|  | M | T | W | T | F | S | S | Notes |
|---|---|---|---|---|---|---|---|---|
| Steps | | | | | | | | |
| Workout | | | | | | | | |
| Water | | | | | | | | |
| Blood Pressure | | | | | | | | |
| Weight/Pulse | | | | | | | | |

Tiny Step for the Week 2 _____

|  | M | T | W | T | F | S | S | Notes |
|---|---|---|---|---|---|---|---|---|
| Steps | | | | | | | | |
| Workout | | | | | | | | |
| Water | | | | | | | | |
| Blood Pressure | | | | | | | | |
| Weight/Pulse | | | | | | | | |

Tiny Step for the Week 3 _____

|  | M | T | W | T | F | S | S | Notes |
|---|---|---|---|---|---|---|---|---|
| Steps | | | | | | | | |
| Workout | | | | | | | | |
| Water | | | | | | | | |
| Blood Pressure | | | | | | | | |
| Weight/Pulse | | | | | | | | |

Tiny Step for the Week 4 _____

|  | M | T | W | T | F | S | S | Notes |
|---|---|---|---|---|---|---|---|---|
| Steps | | | | | | | | |
| Workout | | | | | | | | |
| Water | | | | | | | | |
| Blood Pressure | | | | | | | | |
| Weight/Pulse | | | | | | | | |

## Monthly Measurements

|  | Current | Change |  | Current | Change |  | Current | Change |
|---|---|---|---|---|---|---|---|---|
| Bust | | | Hips | | | BMI | | |
| Waist | | | Thigh | | | BF | | |
| Abdomen | | | Arm | | | Other | | |

# Notes and Reflections

_____

_____

_____

_____

_____

_____

_____

_____

_____

_____

_____

_____

_____

_____

_____

_____

_____

_____

_____

_____

_____

_____

## My Wellness Tracker

Month of _____

3 Month Goal _____

Goal for the Month _____

Tiny Step for the Week 1 _____

|  | M | T | W | T | F | S | S | Notes |
|---|---|---|---|---|---|---|---|---|
| Steps |  |  |  |  |  |  |  |  |
| Workout |  |  |  |  |  |  |  |  |
| Water |  |  |  |  |  |  |  |  |
| Blood Pressure |  |  |  |  |  |  |  |  |
| Weight/Pulse |  |  |  |  |  |  |  |  |

Tiny Step for the Week 2 _____

|  | M | T | W | T | F | S | S | Notes |
|---|---|---|---|---|---|---|---|---|
| Steps |  |  |  |  |  |  |  |  |
| Workout |  |  |  |  |  |  |  |  |
| Water |  |  |  |  |  |  |  |  |
| Blood Pressure |  |  |  |  |  |  |  |  |
| Weight/Pulse |  |  |  |  |  |  |  |  |

Tiny Step for the Week 3 _____

|  | M | T | W | T | F | S | S | Notes |
|---|---|---|---|---|---|---|---|---|
| Steps |  |  |  |  |  |  |  |  |
| Workout |  |  |  |  |  |  |  |  |
| Water |  |  |  |  |  |  |  |  |
| Blood Pressure |  |  |  |  |  |  |  |  |
| Weight/Pulse |  |  |  |  |  |  |  |  |

Tiny Step for the Week 4 _____

|  | M | T | W | T | F | S | S | Notes |
|---|---|---|---|---|---|---|---|---|
| Steps |  |  |  |  |  |  |  |  |
| Workout |  |  |  |  |  |  |  |  |
| Water |  |  |  |  |  |  |  |  |
| Blood Pressure |  |  |  |  |  |  |  |  |
| Weight/Pulse |  |  |  |  |  |  |  |  |

### Monthly Measurements

|  | Current | Change |  | Current | Change |  | Current | Change |
|---|---|---|---|---|---|---|---|---|
| Bust |  |  | Hips |  |  | BMI |  |  |
| Waist |  |  | Thigh |  |  | BF |  |  |
| Abdomen |  |  | Arm |  |  | Other |  |  |

# Notes and Reflections

## My Wellness Tracker

Month of _____

3 Month Goal _____

Goal for the Month _____

Tiny Step for the Week 1 _____

|  | M | T | W | T | F | S | S | Notes |
|---|---|---|---|---|---|---|---|---|
| Steps |  |  |  |  |  |  |  |  |
| Workout |  |  |  |  |  |  |  |  |
| Water |  |  |  |  |  |  |  |  |
| Blood Pressure |  |  |  |  |  |  |  |  |
| Weight/Pulse |  |  |  |  |  |  |  |  |

Tiny Step for the Week 2 _____

|  | M | T | W | T | F | S | S | Notes |
|---|---|---|---|---|---|---|---|---|
| Steps |  |  |  |  |  |  |  |  |
| Workout |  |  |  |  |  |  |  |  |
| Water |  |  |  |  |  |  |  |  |
| Blood Pressure |  |  |  |  |  |  |  |  |
| Weight/Pulse |  |  |  |  |  |  |  |  |

Tiny Step for the Week 3 _____

|  | M | T | W | T | F | S | S | Notes |
|---|---|---|---|---|---|---|---|---|
| Steps |  |  |  |  |  |  |  |  |
| Workout |  |  |  |  |  |  |  |  |
| Water |  |  |  |  |  |  |  |  |
| Blood Pressure |  |  |  |  |  |  |  |  |
| Weight/Pulse |  |  |  |  |  |  |  |  |

Tiny Step for the Week 4 _____

|  | M | T | W | T | F | S | S | Notes |
|---|---|---|---|---|---|---|---|---|
| Steps |  |  |  |  |  |  |  |  |
| Workout |  |  |  |  |  |  |  |  |
| Water |  |  |  |  |  |  |  |  |
| Blood Pressure |  |  |  |  |  |  |  |  |
| Weight/Pulse |  |  |  |  |  |  |  |  |

### Monthly Measurements

|  | Current | Change |  | Current | Change |  | Current | Change |
|---|---|---|---|---|---|---|---|---|
| Bust |  |  | Hips |  |  | BMI |  |  |
| Waist |  |  | Thigh |  |  | BF |  |  |
| Abdomen |  |  | Arm |  |  | Other |  |  |

# Notes and Reflections

# MY FAVORITES/PREFERNCES

| | | | |
|---|---|---|---|
| **Friends** | | | |
| **Pets/animals** | | | |
| **Collectibles** | | | |
| **Games/Hobbies** | | | |
| **TV Shows** | | | |
| **Songs** | | | |
| **Foods** | | | |
| **Books** | | | |
| **Movies** | | | |
| **Websites** | | | |
| **Foods I don't like** | | | |
| **Things I do to relax** | | | |
| **I need help with** | | | |
| **Things I need others to do for me** | | | |
| **More notes** | | | |

# Notes and Reflections

_____
_____
_____
_____
_____
_____
_____
_____
_____
_____
_____
_____
_____
_____
_____
_____
_____
_____
_____
_____
_____
_____
_____

# MY FAMILY SUPPORT RESOURCES

## NAME OF SUPPORT GROUP / ORGANIZATION

_____

Contact Person First and Last Name_____

Organization Address _____

City _____ State _____ Zip Code _____

Contact Phone # (_____) _____ Fax # (_____) _____

Organization Phone # (_____) _____Organization Fax # (_____)_____

Contact Email Address _____

Organization Website _____

## NAME OF RELIGIOUS ORGANIZATION OR PLACE OF WORSHIP

_____

Contact Person First and Last Name_____

Organization Address _____

City _____ State _____ Zip Code _____

Contact Phone # (_____) _____ Fax # (_____) _____

Organization Phone # (_____) _____Organization Fax # (_____)_____

Contact Email Address _____

Organization Website _____
____

# MY FAMILY SUPPORT RESOURCES

## NAME OF COUSELING SERVICE

_____

Contact Person First and Last Name_____

Organization Address_____

City _____ State _____ Zip Code _____

Contact Phone # (_____) _____ Fax # (_____) _____

 Organization Phone # (_____) _____Organization  Fax # (_____)_____

Contact Email Address _____

Organization Website _____

## NAME OF OTHER SUPPORT GROUP / ORGANIZATION

_____

Contact Person First and Last Name_____

Organization Address_____

City _____ State _____ Zip Code _____

Contact Phone # (_____) _____ Fax # (_____) _____

 Organization Phone # (_____) _____Organization  Fax # (_____)_____

Contact Email Address_____

Organization Website _____

_____

# Section 2
# Calendars
# Yearly
# &
# Quarterly

**2022 Yearly Calendar**
**2022 Quarterly Calendars**
**2023 Yearly Calendar**
**2023 Quarterly Calendars**

### JANUARY

| Su | M | Tu | W | Th | F | Sa |
|---|---|---|---|---|---|---|
| | | | | | | 1 |
| 2 | 3 | 4 | 5 | 6 | 7 | 8 |
| 9 | 10 | 11 | 12 | 13 | 14 | 15 |
| 16 | 17 | 18 | 19 | 20 | 21 | 22 |
| 23 | 24 | 25 | 26 | 27 | 28 | 29 |
| 30 | 31 | | | | | |

January 1 New Year's Day

January 17 Martin Luther King Jr. Day

### FEBRUARY

| Su | M | Tu | W | Th | F | Sa |
|---|---|---|---|---|---|---|
| | | 1 | 2 | 3 | 4 | 5 |
| 6 | 7 | 8 | 9 | 10 | 11 | 12 |
| 13 | 14 | 15 | 16 | 17 | 18 | 19 |
| 20 | 21 | 22 | 23 | 24 | 25 | 26 |
| 27 | 28 | | | | | |

February 14 Valentine's Day

February 21 Presidents' Day

### MARCH

| Su | M | Tu | W | Th | F | Sa |
|---|---|---|---|---|---|---|
| | | 1 | 2 | 3 | 4 | 5 |
| 6 | 7 | 8 | 9 | 10 | 11 | 12 |
| 13 | 14 | 15 | 16 | 17 | 18 | 19 |
| 20 | 21 | 22 | 23 | 24 | 25 | 26 |
| 27 | 28 | 29 | 30 | 31 | | |

March 17 St. Patrick's Day

### APRIL

| Su | M | Tu | W | Th | F | Sa |
|---|---|---|---|---|---|---|
| | | | | | 1 | 2 |
| 3 | 4 | 5 | 6 | 7 | 8 | 9 |
| 10 | 11 | 12 | 13 | 14 | 15 | 16 |
| 17 | 18 | 19 | 20 | 21 | 22 | 23 |
| 24 | 25 | 26 | 27 | 28 | 29 | 30 |

April 17 Easter Sunday

April 18 Tax Day

### MAY

| Su | M | Tu | W | Th | F | Sa |
|---|---|---|---|---|---|---|
| 1 | 2 | 3 | 4 | 5 | 6 | 7 |
| 8 | 9 | 10 | 11 | 12 | 13 | 14 |
| 15 | 16 | 17 | 18 | 19 | 20 | 21 |
| 22 | 23 | 24 | 25 | 26 | 27 | 28 |
| 29 | 30 | 31 | | | | |

May 8 Mother's Day

May 30 Memorial Day

### JUNE

| Su | M | Tu | W | Th | F | Sa |
|---|---|---|---|---|---|---|
| | | | 1 | 2 | 3 | 4 |
| 5 | 6 | 7 | 8 | 9 | 10 | 11 |
| 12 | 13 | 14 | 15 | 16 | 17 | 18 |
| 19 | 20 | 21 | 22 | 23 | 24 | 25 |
| 26 | 27 | 28 | 29 | 30 | | |

June 19 Father's Day

June 19 Juneteenth (day off 20th)

### JULY

| Su | M | Tu | W | Th | F | Sa |
|---|---|---|---|---|---|---|
| | | | | | 1 | 2 |
| 3 | 4 | 5 | 6 | 7 | 8 | 9 |
| 10 | 11 | 12 | 13 | 14 | 15 | 16 |
| 17 | 18 | 19 | 20 | 21 | 22 | 23 |
| 24 | 25 | 26 | 27 | 28 | 29 | 30 |
| 31 | | | | | | |

July 4 Independence Day

### AUGUST

| Su | M | Tu | W | Th | F | Sa |
|---|---|---|---|---|---|---|
| | 1 | 2 | 3 | 4 | 5 | 6 |
| 7 | 8 | 9 | 10 | 11 | 12 | 13 |
| 14 | 15 | 16 | 17 | 18 | 19 | 20 |
| 21 | 22 | 23 | 24 | 25 | 26 | 27 |
| 28 | 29 | 30 | 31 | | | |

### SEPTEMBER

| Su | M | Tu | W | Th | F | Sa |
|---|---|---|---|---|---|---|
| | | | | 1 | 2 | 3 |
| 4 | 5 | 6 | 7 | 8 | 9 | 10 |
| 11 | 12 | 13 | 14 | 15 | 16 | 17 |
| 18 | 19 | 20 | 21 | 22 | 23 | 24 |
| 25 | 26 | 27 | 28 | 29 | 30 | |

September 5 Labor Day

### OCTOBER

| Su | M | Tu | W | Th | F | Sa |
|---|---|---|---|---|---|---|
| | | | | | | 1 |
| 2 | 3 | 4 | 5 | 6 | 7 | 8 |
| 9 | 10 | 11 | 12 | 13 | 14 | 15 |
| 16 | 17 | 18 | 19 | 20 | 21 | 22 |
| 23 | 24 | 25 | 26 | 27 | 28 | 29 |
| 30 | 31 | | | | | |

October 10 Columbus Day
October 31 Halloween

### NOVEMBER

| Su | M | Tu | W | Th | F | Sa |
|---|---|---|---|---|---|---|
| | | 1 | 2 | 3 | 4 | 5 |
| 6 | 7 | 8 | 9 | 10 | 11 | 12 |
| 13 | 14 | 15 | 16 | 17 | 18 | 19 |
| 20 | 21 | 22 | 23 | 24 | 25 | 26 |
| 27 | 28 | 29 | 30 | | | |

November 11 Veterans' Day
November 24 Thanksgiving Day

### DECEMBER

| Su | M | Tu | W | Th | F | Sa |
|---|---|---|---|---|---|---|
| | | | | 1 | 2 | 3 |
| 4 | 5 | 6 | 7 | 8 | 9 | 10 |
| 11 | 12 | 13 | 14 | 15 | 16 | 17 |
| 18 | 19 | 20 | 21 | 22 | 23 | 24 |
| 25 | 26 | 27 | 28 | 29 | 30 | 31 |

December 25 Christmas Day (day off 26th)
December 31 New Year's Eve

| | SUN | MON | TUE | WED | THU | FRI | SAT | NOTES |
|---|---|---|---|---|---|---|---|---|
| **JANUARY 2022** | | | | | | | 1 | |
| | 2 | 3 | 4 | 5 | 6 | 7 | 8 | |
| | 9 | 10 | 11 | 12 | 13 | 14 | 15 | |
| | 16 | 17 | 18 | 19 | 20 | 21 | 22 | |
| | 23 | 24 | 25 | 26 | 27 | 28 | 29 | |
| | 30 | 31 | | | | | | |
| **FEBRUARY 2022** | | | 1 | 2 | 3 | 4 | 5 | |
| | 6 | 7 | 8 | 9 | 10 | 11 | 12 | |
| | 13 | 14 | 15 | 16 | 17 | 18 | 19 | |
| | 20 | 21 | 22 | 23 | 24 | 25 | 26 | |
| | 27 | 28 | | | | | | |
| | | | | | | | | |
| **MARCH 2022** | | | 1 | 2 | 3 | 4 | 5 | |
| | 6 | 7 | 8 | 9 | 10 | 11 | 12 | |
| | 13 | 14 | 15 | 16 | 17 | 18 | 19 | |
| | 20 | 21 | 22 | 23 | 24 | 25 | 26 | |
| | 27 | 28 | | | | | | |

Holidays: January 1 New Year's Day      17 Martin Luther King, Jr. Day
February 14 Valentine's Day   21 President's Day

| | SUN | MON | TUE | WED | THU | FRI | SAT | NOTES |
|---|---|---|---|---|---|---|---|---|
| **APRIL 2022** | | | | | | 1 | 2 | |
| | 3 | 4 | 5 | 6 | 7 | 8 | 9 | |
| | 10 | 11 | 12 | 13 | 14 | 15 | 16 | |
| | 17 | 18 | 19 | 20 | 21 | 22 | 23 | |
| | 24 | 25 | 26 | 27 | 28 | 29 | 30 | |
| | | | | | | | | |
| **MAY 2022** | 1 | 2 | 3 | 4 | 5 | 6 | 7 | |
| | 8 | 9 | 10 | 11 | 12 | 13 | 14 | |
| | 14 | 15 | 16 | 17 | 18 | 19 | 21 | |
| | 22 | 23 | 24 | 25 | 26 | 27 | 28 | |
| | 29 | 30 | 31 | | | | | |
| | | | | | | | | |
| **JUNE 2022** | | | | 1 | 2 | 3 | 4 | |
| | 5 | 6 | 7 | 8 | 9 | 10 | 11 | |
| | 12 | 13 | 14 | 15 | 16 | 17 | 18 | |
| | 19 | 20 | 21 | 22 | 23 | 24 | 25 | |
| | 26 | 27 | 28 | 29 | 30 | | | |

Holidays: May 8 Mother's Day     30 Memorial Day
June 19 Father's Day

| | SUN | MON | TUE | WED | THU | FRI | SAT | NOTES |
|---|---|---|---|---|---|---|---|---|
| **JULY 2022** | | | | | | 1 | 2 | |
| | 3 | 4 | 5 | 6 | 7 | 8 | 9 | |
| | 10 | 11 | 12 | 13 | 14 | 15 | 16 | |
| | 17 | 18 | 19 | 20 | 21 | 22 | 23 | |
| | 24 | 25 | 26 | 27 | 28 | 29 | 30 | |
| | 31 | | | | | | | |
| **AUGUST 2022** | | 1 | 2 | 3 | 4 | 5 | 6 | |
| | 7 | 8 | 9 | 10 | 11 | 12 | 13 | |
| | 14 | 15 | 16 | 17 | 18 | 19 | 20 | |
| | 21 | 22 | 23 | 24 | 25 | 26 | 27 | |
| | 28 | 29 | 30 | 31 | | | | |
| | | | | | | | | |
| **SEPTEMBER 2022** | | | | | 1 | 2 | 3 | |
| | 4 | 5 | 6 | 7 | 8 | 9 | 10 | |
| | 11 | 12 | 13 | 14 | 15 | 16 | 17 | |
| | 18 | 19 | 20 | 21 | 22 | 23 | 24 | |
| | 25 | 26 | 27 | 28 | 29 | 30 | | |

Holidays: July 4 Independence Day
September 5 Labor Day

| | SUN | MON | TUE | WED | THU | FRI | SAT | NOTES |
|---|---|---|---|---|---|---|---|---|
| **OCTOBER 2022** | | | | | | | 1 | |
| | 2 | 3 | 4 | 5 | 6 | 7 | 8 | |
| | 9 | 10 | 11 | 12 | 13 | 14 | 15 | |
| | 16 | 17 | 18 | 19 | 20 | 21 | 22 | |
| | 23 | 24 | 25 | 26 | 27 | 28 | 29 | |
| | 30 | 31 | | | | | | |
| **NOVEMBER 2022** | | | 1 | 2 | 3 | 4 | 5 | |
| | 6 | 7 | 8 | 9 | 10 | 11 | 12 | |
| | 13 | 14 | 15 | 16 | 17 | 18 | 19 | |
| | 20 | 21 | 22 | 23 | 24 | 25 | 26 | |
| | 27 | 28 | 29 | 30 | | | | |
| | | | | | | | | |
| **DECEMBER 2022** | | | | | 1 | 2 | 3 | |
| | 4 | 5 | 6 | 7 | 8 | 9 | 10 | |
| | 11 | 12 | 13 | 14 | 15 | 16 | 17 | |
| | 18 | 19 | 20 | 21 | 22 | 23 | 24 | |
| | 25 | 26 | 27 | 28 | 29 | 30 | 31 | |

Holidays: October 10 Columbus Day   31 Halloween
November 11 Veterans Day   24 Thanksgiving
December 25 Christmas

## JANUARY

| Su | M | Tu | W | Th | F | Sa |
|---|---|---|---|---|---|---|
| 1 | 2 | 3 | 4 | 5 | 6 | 7 |
| 8 | 9 | 10 | 11 | 12 | 13 | 14 |
| 15 | 16 | 17 | 18 | 19 | 20 | 21 |
| 22 | 23 | 24 | 25 | 26 | 27 | 28 |
| 29 | 30 | 31 | | | | |

January 1 New Year's Day(day off 2nd)
January 16 Martin Luther King Jr. Day

## FEBRUARY

| Su | M | Tu | W | Th | F | Sa |
|---|---|---|---|---|---|---|
| | | | 1 | 2 | 3 | 4 |
| 5 | 6 | 7 | 8 | 9 | 10 | 11 |
| 12 | 13 | 14 | 15 | 16 | 17 | 18 |
| 19 | 20 | 21 | 22 | 23 | 24 | 25 |
| 26 | 27 | 28 | | | | |

February 14 Valentine's Day
February 20 Presidents' Day

## MARCH

| Su | M | Tu | W | Th | F | Sa |
|---|---|---|---|---|---|---|
| | | | 1 | 2 | 3 | 4 |
| 5 | 6 | 7 | 8 | 9 | 10 | 11 |
| 12 | 13 | 14 | 15 | 16 | 17 | 18 |
| 19 | 20 | 21 | 22 | 23 | 24 | 25 |
| 26 | 27 | 28 | 29 | 30 | 31 | |

March 17 St. Patrick's Day

## APRIL

| Su | M | Tu | W | Th | F | Sa |
|---|---|---|---|---|---|---|
| | | | | | | 1 |
| 2 | 3 | 4 | 5 | 6 | 7 | 8 |
| 9 | 10 | 11 | 12 | 13 | 14 | 15 |
| 16 | 17 | 18 | 19 | 20 | 21 | 22 |
| 23 | 24 | 25 | 26 | 27 | 28 | 29 |
| 30 | | | | | | |

April 9 Easter Sunday
April 18 Tax Day

## MAY

| Su | M | Tu | W | Th | F | Sa |
|---|---|---|---|---|---|---|
| | 1 | 2 | 3 | 4 | 5 | 6 |
| 7 | 8 | 9 | 10 | 11 | 12 | 13 |
| 14 | 15 | 16 | 17 | 18 | 19 | 20 |
| 21 | 22 | 23 | 24 | 25 | 26 | 27 |
| 28 | 29 | 30 | 31 | | | |

May 14 Mother's Day
May 29 Memorial Day

## JUNE

| Su | M | Tu | W | Th | F | Sa |
|---|---|---|---|---|---|---|
| | | | | 1 | 2 | 3 |
| 4 | 5 | 6 | 7 | 8 | 9 | 10 |
| 11 | 12 | 13 | 14 | 15 | 16 | 17 |
| 18 | 19 | 20 | 21 | 22 | 23 | 24 |
| 25 | 26 | 27 | 28 | 29 | 30 | |

June 18 Father's Day
June 19 Juneteenth

## JULY

| Su | M | Tu | W | Th | F | Sa |
|---|---|---|---|---|---|---|
| | | | | | | 1 |
| 2 | 3 | 4 | 5 | 6 | 7 | 8 |
| 9 | 10 | 11 | 12 | 13 | 14 | 15 |
| 16 | 17 | 18 | 19 | 20 | 21 | 22 |
| 23 | 24 | 25 | 26 | 27 | 28 | 29 |
| 30 | 31 | | | | | |

July 4 Independence Day

## AUGUST

| Su | M | Tu | W | Th | F | Sa |
|---|---|---|---|---|---|---|
| | | 1 | 2 | 3 | 4 | 5 |
| 6 | 7 | 8 | 9 | 10 | 11 | 12 |
| 13 | 14 | 15 | 16 | 17 | 18 | 19 |
| 20 | 21 | 22 | 23 | 24 | 25 | 26 |
| 27 | 28 | 29 | 30 | 31 | | |

## SEPTEMBER

| Su | M | Tu | W | Th | F | Sa |
|---|---|---|---|---|---|---|
| | | | | | 1 | 2 |
| 3 | 4 | 5 | 6 | 7 | 8 | 9 |
| 10 | 11 | 12 | 13 | 14 | 15 | 16 |
| 17 | 18 | 19 | 20 | 21 | 22 | 23 |
| 24 | 25 | 26 | 27 | 28 | 29 | 30 |

September 4 Labor Day

## OCTOBER

| Su | M | Tu | W | Th | F | Sa |
|---|---|---|---|---|---|---|
| 1 | 2 | 3 | 4 | 5 | 6 | 7 |
| 8 | 9 | 10 | 11 | 12 | 13 | 14 |
| 15 | 16 | 17 | 18 | 19 | 20 | 21 |
| 22 | 23 | 24 | 25 | 26 | 27 | 28 |
| 29 | 30 | 31 | | | | |

October 9 Columbus Day
October 31 Halloween

## NOVEMBER

| Su | M | Tu | W | Th | F | Sa |
|---|---|---|---|---|---|---|
| | | | 1 | 2 | 3 | 4 |
| 5 | 6 | 7 | 8 | 9 | 10 | 11 |
| 12 | 13 | 14 | 15 | 16 | 17 | 18 |
| 19 | 20 | 21 | 22 | 23 | 24 | 25 |
| 26 | 27 | 28 | 29 | 30 | | |

November 11 Veterans' Day (off 10th)
November 23 Thanksgiving Day

## DECEMBER

| Su | M | Tu | W | Th | F | Sa |
|---|---|---|---|---|---|---|
| | | | | | 1 | 2 |
| 3 | 4 | 5 | 6 | 7 | 8 | 9 |
| 10 | 11 | 12 | 13 | 14 | 15 | 16 |
| 17 | 18 | 19 | 20 | 21 | 22 | 23 |
| 24 | 25 | 26 | 27 | 28 | 29 | 30 |
| 31 | | | | | | |

December 25 Christmas Day
December 31 New Year's Eve

| | SUN | MON | TUE | WED | THU | FRI | SAT | NOTES |
|---|---|---|---|---|---|---|---|---|
| **JANUARY 2023** | | | | | | | | |
| | 1 | 2 | 3 | 4 | 5 | 6 | 7 | |
| | 8 | 9 | 10 | 11 | 12 | 13 | 14 | |
| | 15 | 16 | 17 | 18 | 10 | 20 | 21 | |
| | 22 | 23 | 24 | 25 | 26 | 27 | 28 | |
| | 29 | 30 | 31 | | | | | |
| **FEBRUARY 2023** | | | | 1 | 2 | 3 | 4 | |
| | 5 | 6 | 7 | 8 | 9 | 10 | 11 | |
| | 12 | 13 | 14 | 15 | 16 | 17 | 18 | |
| | 19 | 20 | 21 | 22 | 23 | 24 | 25 | |
| | 26 | 27 | 28 | | | | | |
| | | | | | | | | |
| **MARCH 2023** | | | | 1 | 2 | 3 | 4 | |
| | 5 | 6 | 7 | 8 | 9 | 10 | 11 | |
| | 12 | 13 | 14 | 15 | 16 | 17 | 18 | |
| | 19 | 20 | 21 | 22 | 23 | 24 | 25 | |
| | 26 | 27 | 28 | 29 | 30 | 31 | | |

Holidays: January 1 New Year's Day    16 Martin Luther King, Jr. Day
February 14 Valentine's Day   20 President's Day

|  | SUN | MON | TUE | WED | THU | FRI | SAT | NOTES |
|---|---|---|---|---|---|---|---|---|
| **APRIL 2023** |  |  |  |  |  |  | 1 |  |
|  | 2 | 3 | 4 | 5 | 6 | 7 | 8 |  |
|  | 9 | 10 | 11 | 12 | 13 | 14 | 15 |  |
|  | 16 | 17 | 18 | 19 | 20 | 21 | 22 |  |
|  | 23 | 24 | 25 | 26 | 27 | 28 | 29 |  |
|  | 30 |  |  |  |  |  |  |  |
| **MAY 2023** |  | 1 | 2 | 3 | 4 | 5 | 6 |  |
|  | 7 | 8 | 9 | 10 | 11 | 12 | 13 |  |
|  | 14 | 15 | 16 | 17 | 18 | 19 | 20 |  |
|  | 21 | 22 | 23 | 24 | 25 | 26 | 27 |  |
|  | 28 | 29 | 30 | 31 |  |  |  |  |
|  |  |  |  |  |  |  |  |  |
| **JUNE 2023** |  |  |  |  | 1 | 2 | 3 |  |
|  | 4 | 5 | 6 | 7 | 8 | 9 | 10 |  |
|  | 11 | 12 | 13 | 14 | 15 | 16 | 17 |  |
|  | 18 | 19 | 20 | 21 | 22 | 23 | 24 |  |
|  | 25 | 26 | 27 | 28 | 29 | 30 |  |  |

Holidays: May 14 Mother's Day     29 Memorial Day
June 18 Father's Day     19 Juneteenth Holiday

| | SUN | MON | TUE | WED | THU | FRI | SAT | NOTES |
|---|---|---|---|---|---|---|---|---|
| **JULY 2023** | | | | | | | 1 | |
| | 2 | 3 | 4 | 5 | 6 | 7 | 8 | |
| | 9 | 10 | 11 | 12 | 13 | 14 | 15 | |
| | 16 | 17 | 18 | 19 | 20 | 21 | 22 | |
| | 23 | 24 | 25 | 26 | 27 | 28 | 29 | |
| | 30 | 31 | | | | | | |
| **AUGUST 2023** | | | 1 | 2 | 3 | 4 | 5 | |
| | 6 | 7 | 8 | 9 | 10 | 11 | 12 | |
| | 13 | 14 | 15 | 16 | 17 | 18 | 19 | |
| | 20 | 21 | 22 | 23 | 24 | 25 | 26 | |
| | 27 | 28 | 29 | 30 | 31 | | | |
| | | | | | | | | |
| **SEPTEMBER 2023** | | | | | | 1 | 2 | |
| | 3 | 4 | 5 | 6 | 7 | 8 | 9 | |
| | 10 | 11 | 12 | 13 | 14 | 15 | 16 | |
| | 17 | 18 | 19 | 20 | 21 | 22 | 23 | |
| | 24 | 25 | 26 | 27 | 28 | 29 | 30 | |
| | Holidays: July 4 Independence Day | | | | | | | |
| | September 4 Labor Day | | | | | | | |

|  | SUN | MON | TUE | WED | THU | FRI | SAT | NOTES |
|---|---|---|---|---|---|---|---|---|
| **OCTOBER 2023** |  |  |  |  |  |  |  |  |
|  | 1 | 2 | 3 | 4 | 5 | 6 | 7 |  |
|  | 8 | 9 | 10 | 11 | 12 | 13 | 14 |  |
|  | 15 | 16 | 17 | 18 | 19 | 20 | 21 |  |
|  | 22 | 23 | 24 | 25 | 26 | 27 | 28 |  |
|  | 29 | 30 | 31 |  |  |  |  |  |
| **NOVEMBER 2023** |  |  |  | 1 | 2 | 3 | 4 |  |
|  | 5 | 6 | 7 | 8 | 9 | 10 | 11 |  |
|  | 12 | 13 | 14 | 15 | 16 | 17 | 18 |  |
|  | 19 | 20 | 21 | 22 | 23 | 24 | 25 |  |
|  | 26 | 27 | 28 | 29 | 30 |  |  |  |
|  |  |  |  |  |  |  |  |  |
| **DECEMBER 2023** |  |  |  |  |  | 1 | 2 |  |
|  | 3 | 4 | 5 | 6 | 7 | 8 | 9 |  |
|  | 10 | 11 | 12 | 13 | 14 | 15 | 16 |  |
|  | 17 | 18 | 19 | 20 | 21 | 22 | 23 |  |
|  | 24/31 | 25 | 26 | 27 | 28 | 29 | 30 |  |

Holidays: October 9 Columbus Day      31 Halloween
November 11 Veterans Day      23 Thanksgiving
December 25 Christmas

# Notes and Reflections

# Section 3
# Doctor Visits with Question Logs

- ❖ **Appointment & Question Logs**
- ❖ **Doctor/Provider Visit Notes (24)**
- ❖ **Equipment Lists**
- ❖ **Supplies List**

# APPOINTMENT & QUESTION LOGS

Write down your questions and problems before you go to see a medical provider. Show this log to your provider during the visit and write down any answers to your questions. Use the DOCTOR'S/PROVIDER'S Visit Note Pages for detailed notes. (see following pages)

| Day/ Month/ Day/ Year/ Time | Provider & Phone Number | Reason seen and care to provide | Questions or problems to discuss | Next appointment Day/Month/ Date/ Year/Time |
|---|---|---|---|---|
| | | | | |
| | | | | |
| | | | | |
| | | | | |
| | | | | |
| | | | | |
| | | | | |
| | | | | |
| | | | | |
| | | | | |
| | | | | |

**REMEMBER TO CALL TO CANCEL OR RESCHEDULE YOUR APPOINTMENT IF YOU CAN'T MAKE IT**

# APPOINTMENT & QUESTION LOGS

Write down your questions and problems before you go to see a medical provider. Show this log to your provider during the visit and write down any answers to your questions. Use the DOCTOR'S/PROVIDER'S Visit Note Pages for detailed notes. (see following pages)

| Day/ Month/ Day/ Year/ Time | Provider & Phone Number | Reason seen and care to provide | Questions or problems to discuss | Next appointment Day/Month/ Date/ Year/Time |
|---|---|---|---|---|
|  |  |  |  |  |
|  |  |  |  |  |
|  |  |  |  |  |
|  |  |  |  |  |
|  |  |  |  |  |
|  |  |  |  |  |
|  |  |  |  |  |
|  |  |  |  |  |
|  |  |  |  |  |
|  |  |  |  |  |
|  |  |  |  |  |

| REMEMBER TO CALL TO CANCEL OR RESCHEDULE YOUR APPOINTMENT IF YOU CAN'T MAKE IT |
|---|

# APPOINTMENT & QUESTION LOGS

Write down your questions and problems before you go to see a medical provider. Show this log to your provider during the visit and write down any answers to your questions. Use the DOCTOR'S/PROVIDER'S Visit Note Pages for detailed notes. (see following pages)

| Day/ Month/ Day/ Year/ Time | Provider & Phone Number | Reason seen and care to provide | Questions or problems to discuss | Next appointment Day/Month/ Date/ Year/Time |
|---|---|---|---|---|
| | | | | |
| | | | | |
| | | | | |
| | | | | |
| | | | | |
| | | | | |
| | | | | |
| | | | | |
| | | | | |
| | | | | |
| | | | | |

**REMEMBER TO CALL TO CANCEL OR RESCHEDULE YOUR APPOINTMENT IF YOU CAN'T MAKE IT**

# APPOINTMENT & QUESTION LOGS

Write down your questions and problems before you go to see a medical provider. Show this log to your provider during the visit and write down any answers to your questions. Use the DOCTOR'S/PROVIDER'S Visit Note Pages for detailed notes. (see following pages)

| Day/ Month/ Day/ Year/ Time | Provider & Phone Number | Reason seen and care to provide | Questions or problems to discuss | Next appointment Day/Month/ Date/ Year/Time |
|---|---|---|---|---|
| | | | | |
| | | | | |
| | | | | |
| | | | | |
| | | | | |
| | | | | |
| | | | | |
| | | | | |
| | | | | |
| | | | | |
| | | | | |

**REMEMBER TO CALL TO CANCEL OR RESCHEDULE YOUR APPOINTMENT IF YOU CAN'T MAKE IT**

# Notes and Reflections

_____
_____
_____
_____
_____
_____
_____
_____
_____
_____
_____
_____
_____
_____
_____
_____
_____
_____
_____
_____
_____
_____

# DOCTOR'S/PROVIDER'S VISIT NOTES

Day/Date of visit_____ Doctor to see _____

Location/Address _____Phone # _____

Directions

_____

_____

Pre-visit instructions?

_____

_____

_____

## BEFORE THE VISIT

Reason for today's visit?

_____

_____

_____

How long has this been going on?

_____

_____

_____

What makes it better or worse?

_____

_____

_____

What have you tried so far?

_____

_____

_____

## NOTES FROM THE VISIT

What is the diagnosis? _____

_____

_____

Are there any tests to do? No ☐ Yes ☐     Any procedures to do? No ☐ Yes ☐

What test/procedure & where?_____

_____

_____

_____

_____

Was a prescription given? No ☐   Yes ☐

What is the medicine and dosage?_____

Are there side effects to this medicine? _____

If no medicine was needed, what should I do? _____

What should I do if symptoms return? _____

Where could I get more information? _____

Notes: BP _____ Pulse _____Weight _____Temperature_____ O₂ ____

_____

_____

_____

Is there going to be a follow up appointment? No ☐   Yes ☐ When? _____

Actions for me to take: _____

| REMEMBER TO CALL TO CANCEL OR RESCHEDULE YOUR APPOINTMENT IF YOU CAN'T MAKE IT |
| --- |

# DOCTOR'S/PROVIDER'S VISIT NOTES

Day/Date of visit_____ Doctor to see _____

Location/Address _____ Phone # _____

Directions

_____

_____

Pre-visit instructions?

_____

_____

_____

## BEFORE THE VISIT

Reason for today's visit?

_____

_____

_____

How long has this been going on?

_____

_____

_____

What makes it better or worse?

_____

_____

_____

What have you tried so far?

_____

_____

_____

## NOTES FROM THE VISIT

What is the diagnosis? _____

_____

_____

_____

Are there any tests to do? No ☐ Yes ☐    Any procedures to do? No ☐ Yes ☐

What test/procedure & where?_____

_____

_____

_____

Was a prescription given? No ☐   Yes ☐

What is the medicine and dosage?_____

Are there side effects to this medicine? _____

If no medicine was needed, what should I do? _____

What should I do if symptoms return? _____

Where could I get more information? _____

Notes: BP _____ Pulse _____Weight _____Temperature_____ O₂____

_____

_____

_____

Is there going to be a follow up appointment? No ☐   Yes ☐ When? _____

Actions for me to take: _____

| REMEMBER TO CALL TO CANCEL OR RESCHEDULE YOUR APPOINTMENT IF YOU CAN'T MAKE IT |
| --- |

# DOCTOR'S/PROVIDER'S VISIT NOTES

Day/Date of visit_____Doctor to see _____

Location/Address _____Phone # _____

Directions

_____

_____

Pre-visit instructions?

_____

_____

_____

## BEFORE THE VISIT

Reason for today's visit?

_____

_____

How long has this been going on?

_____

_____

What makes it better or worse?

_____

_____

What have you tried so far?

_____

_____

_____

## NOTES FROM THE VISIT

What is the diagnosis? _____

_____

_____

_____

Are there any tests to do? No ☐ Yes ☐          Any procedures to do? No ☐ Yes ☐

What test/procedure & where?_____

_____

_____

_____

Was a prescription given? No ☐   Yes ☐

What is the medicine and dosage?_____

Are there side effects to this medicine? _____

If no medicine was needed, what should I do? _____

What should I do if symptoms return? _____

Where could I get more information? _____

Notes: BP _____ Pulse _____Weight _____Temperature_____ O$_2$ ____

_____

_____

_____

Is there going to be a follow up appointment? No ☐   Yes ☐ When? _____

Actions for me to take: _____

**REMEMBER TO CALL TO CANCEL OR RESCHEDULE YOUR APPOINTMENT IF YOU CAN'T MAKE IT**

# DOCTOR'S/PROVIDER'S VISIT NOTES

Day/Date of visit_____Doctor to see _____

Location/Address _____Phone # _____

Directions

_____

_____

Pre-visit instructions?

_____

_____

_____

## BEFORE THE VISIT

Reason for today's visit?

_____

_____

How long has this been going on?

_____

_____

What makes it better or worse?

_____

_____

What have you tried so far?

_____

_____

_____

## NOTES FROM THE VISIT

What is the diagnosis? _____

_____

_____

_____

Are there any tests to do? No ☐ Yes ☐         Any procedures to do? No ☐ Yes ☐

What test/procedure & where?_____

_____

_____

_____

Was a prescription given? No ☐   Yes ☐

What is the medicine and dosage?_____

Are there side effects to this medicine? _____

If no medicine was needed, what should I do? _____

What should I do if symptoms return? _____

Where could I get more information? _____

Notes: BP _____ Pulse _____Weight _____Temperature_____ O$_2$ ____

_____

_____

_____

Is there going to be a follow up appointment? No ☐   Yes ☐ When? _____

Actions for me to take: _____

| REMEMBER TO CALL TO CANCEL OR RESCHEDULE YOUR APPOINTMENT IF YOU CAN'T MAKE IT |
| --- |

# DOCTOR'S/PROVIDER'S VISIT NOTES

Day/Date of visit_____Doctor to see _____

Location/Address _____Phone # _____

Directions

_____

_____

Pre-visit instructions?

_____

_____

_____

Reason for today's visit?

_____

_____

_____

How long has this been going on?

_____

_____

_____

What makes it better or worse?

_____

_____

_____

What have you tried so far?

_____

_____

_____

What is the diagnosis? _____

_____

_____

_____

Are there any tests to do? No ☐ Yes ☐      Any procedures to do? No ☐ Yes ☐

What test/procedure & where?_____

_____

_____

_____

Are there any tests to do? No ☐ Yes ☐      Any procedures to do? No ☐ Yes ☐

What test/procedure & where?_____

Was a prescription given? No ☐   Yes ☐

What is the medicine and dosage?_____

Are there side effects to this medicine? _____

If no medicine was needed, what should I do? _____

What should I do if symptoms return? _____

Where could I get more information? _____

Notes: BP _____ Pulse _____Weight _____Temperature_____ O₂ _____

_____

_____

_____

Is there going to be a follow up appointment? No ☐   Yes ☐ When? _____

Actions for me to take: _____

**REMEMBER TO CALL TO CANCEL OR RESCHEDULE YOUR APPOINTMENT IF YOU CAN'T MAKE IT**

# DOCTOR'S/PROVIDER'S VISIT NOTES

Day/Date of visit_____Doctor to see _____

Location/Address _____Phone # _____

Directions

_____

_____

Pre-visit instructions?

_____

_____

_____

## BEFORE THE VISIT

Reason for today's visit?

_____

_____

_____

How long has this been going on?

_____

_____

_____

What makes it better or worse?

_____

_____

_____

What have you tried so far?

_____

_____

_____

What is the diagnosis? _____

_____

_____

_____

Are there any tests to do? No ☐ Yes ☐          Any procedures to do? No ☐ Yes ☐

What test/procedure & where?_____

_____

_____

_____

Was a prescription given? No ☐   Yes ☐

What is the medicine and dosage?_____

Are there side effects to this medicine? _____

If no medicine was needed, what should I do? _____

What should I do if symptoms return? _____

Where could I get more information? _____

Notes: BP _____ Pulse _____Weight _____Temperature_____ O$_2$ _____

_____

_____

_____

Is there going to be a follow up appointment? No ☐   Yes ☐ When? _____

Actions for me to take: _____

REMEMBER TO CALL TO CANCEL OR RESCHEDULE YOUR APPOINTMENT IF YOU CAN'T MAKE IT

# DOCTOR'S/PROVIDER'S VISIT NOTES

Day/Date of visit_____ Doctor to see _____

Location/Address _____ Phone # _____

Directions

_____

_____

Pre-visit instructions?

_____

_____

## BEFORE THE VISIT

Reason for today's visit?

_____

_____

How long has this been going on?

_____

_____

What makes it better or worse?

_____

_____

What have you tried so far?

_____

_____

_____

## NOTES FROM THE VISIT

What is the diagnosis? _____

_____

_____

_____

Are there any tests to do? No ☐ Yes ☐     Any procedures to do? No ☐ Yes ☐

What test/procedure & where?_____

_____

_____

_____

Was a prescription given? No ☐   Yes ☐

What is the medicine and dosage?_____

Are there side effects to this medicine? _____

If no medicine was needed, what should I do? _____

What should I do if symptoms return? _____

Where could I get more information? _____

Notes: BP _____ Pulse _____Weight _____Temperature_____ O$_2$ _____

_____

_____

_____

Is there going to be a follow up appointment? No ☐   Yes ☐ When? _____

Actions for me to take: _____

REMEMBER TO CALL TO CANCEL OR RESCHEDULE YOUR APPOINTMENT IF YOU CAN'T MAKE IT

# DOCTOR'S/PROVIDER'S VISIT NOTES

Day/Date of visit _____ Doctor to see _____

Location/Address _____ Phone # _____

Directions

_____

_____

Pre-visit instructions?

_____

_____

_____

## BEFORE THE VISIT

Reason for today's visit?

_____

_____

_____

How long has this been going on?

_____

_____

_____

What makes it better or worse?

_____

_____

_____

What have you tried so far?

_____

_____

_____

## NOTES FROM THE VISIT

What is the diagnosis? _____

_____

_____

_____

Are there any tests to do? No ☐ Yes ☐    Any procedures to do? No ☐ Yes ☐

What test/procedure & where?_____

_____

_____

_____

Was a prescription given? No ☐ Yes ☐

What is the medicine and dosage?_____

Are there side effects to this medicine? _____

If no medicine was needed, what should I do? _____

What should I do if symptoms return? _____

Where could I get more information? _____

Notes: BP _____ Pulse _____Weight _____Temperature_____ O$_2$ _____

_____

_____

_____

Is there going to be a follow up appointment? No ☐ Yes ☐ When? _____

Actions for me to take: _____

> **REMEMBER TO CALL TO CANCEL OR RESCHEDULE YOUR APPOINTMENT IF YOU CAN'T MAKE IT**

# DOCTOR'S/PROVIDER'S VISIT NOTES

Day/Date of visit _____ Doctor to see _____

Location/Address _____ Phone # _____

Directions

_____

_____

Pre-visit instructions?

_____

_____

_____

## BEFORE THE VISIT

Reason for today's visit?

_____

_____

_____

How long has this been going on?

_____

_____

_____

What makes it better or worse?

_____

_____

_____

What have you tried so far?

_____

_____

_____

## NOTES FROM THE VISIT

What is the diagnosis? _____

_____

_____

_____

Are there any tests to do? No ☐ Yes ☐        Any procedures to do? No ☐ Yes ☐

What test/procedure & where?_____

_____

_____

_____

Was a prescription given? No ☐   Yes ☐

What is the medicine and dosage?_____

Are there side effects to this medicine? _____

If no medicine was needed, what should I do? _____

What should I do if symptoms return? _____

Where could I get more information? _____

Notes: BP _____ Pulse _____Weight _____Temperature_____ $O_2$ ____

_____

_____

_____

Is there going to be a follow up appointment? No ☐   Yes ☐ When? _____

Actions for me to take: _____

**REMEMBER TO CALL TO CANCEL OR RESCHEDULE YOUR APPOINTMENT IF YOU CAN'T MAKE IT**

# DOCTOR'S/PROVIDER'S VISIT NOTES

Day/Date of visit_____ Doctor to see _____

Location/Address _____Phone # _____

Directions

_____

_____

Pre-visit instructions?

_____

_____

_____

## BEFORE THE VISIT

Reason for today's visit?

_____

_____

_____

How long has this been going on?

_____

_____

_____

What makes it better or worse?

_____

_____

_____

What have you tried so far?

_____

_____

_____

## NOTES FROM THE VISIT

What is the diagnosis? _____

_____

_____

_____

Are there any tests to do? No ☐ Yes ☐        Any procedures to do? No ☐ Yes ☐

What test/procedure & where?_____

_____

_____

_____

Was a prescription given? No ☐   Yes ☐

What is the medicine and dosage?_____

Are there side effects to this medicine? _____

If no medicine was needed, what should I do? _____

What should I do if symptoms return? _____

Where could I get more information? _____

Notes: BP _____ Pulse _____Weight _____Temperature_____ O$_2$ ____

_____

_____

_____

Is there going to be a follow up appointment? No ☐   Yes ☐ When? _____

Actions for me to take: _____

REMEMBER TO CALL TO CANCEL OR RESCHEDULE YOUR APPOINTMENT IF YOU CAN'T MAKE IT

# DOCTOR'S/PROVIDER'S VISIT NOTES

Day/Date of visit_____ Doctor to see _____

Location/Address _____ Phone # _____

Directions

_____

_____

Pre-visit instructions?

_____

_____

_____

## BEFORE THE VISIT

Reason for today's visit?

_____

_____

How long has this been going on?

_____

_____

What makes it better or worse?

_____

_____

What have you tried so far?

_____

_____

_____

## NOTES FROM THE VISIT

What is the diagnosis? _____

_____

_____

_____

Are there any tests to do? No ☐ Yes ☐          Any procedures to do? No ☐ Yes ☐

What test/procedure & where?_____

_____

_____

_____

Was a prescription given? No ☐   Yes ☐

What is the medicine and dosage?_____

Are there side effects to this medicine? _____

If no medicine was needed, what should I do? _____

What should I do if symptoms return? _____

Where could I get more information? _____

Notes: BP _____ Pulse _____Weight _____Temperature_____ O$_2$ _____

_____

_____

_____

Is there going to be a follow up appointment? No ☐   Yes ☐ When? _____

Actions for me to take: _____

**REMEMBER TO CALL TO CANCEL OR RESCHEDULE YOUR APPOINTMENT IF YOU CAN'T MAKE IT**

# DOCTOR'S/PROVIDER'S VISIT NOTES

Day/Date of visit_____Doctor to see _____

Location/Address _____Phone # _____

Directions

_____

_____

Pre-visit instructions?

_____

_____

_____

## BEFORE THE VISIT

Reason for today's visit?

_____

_____

_____

How long has this been going on?

_____

_____

_____

What makes it better or worse?

_____

_____

_____

What have you tried so far?

_____

_____

_____

## NOTES FROM THE VISIT

What is the diagnosis? _____

_____

_____

_____

Are there any tests to do? No ☐ Yes ☐        Any procedures to do? No ☐ Yes ☐

What test/procedure & where?_____

_____

_____

_____

Was a prescription given? No ☐   Yes ☐

What is the medicine and dosage?_____

Are there side effects to this medicine? _____

If no medicine was needed, what should I do? _____

What should I do if symptoms return? _____

Where could I get more information? _____

Notes: BP _____ Pulse _____Weight _____Temperature_____ O$_2$_____

_____

_____

_____

Is there going to be a follow up appointment? No ☐   Yes ☐ When? _____

Actions for me to take: _____

| REMEMBER TO CALL TO CANCEL OR RESCHEDULE YOUR APPOINTMENT IF YOU CAN'T MAKE IT |
| --- |

# DOCTOR'S/PROVIDER'S VISIT NOTES

Day/Date of visit_____Doctor to see _____

Location/Address _____Phone # _____

Directions

_____

_____

Pre-visit instructions?

_____

_____

_____

## BEFORE THE VISIT

Reason for today's visit?

_____

_____

_____

How long has this been going on?

_____

_____

_____

What makes it better or worse?

_____

_____

_____

What have you tried so far?

_____

_____

_____

## NOTES FROM THE VISIT

What is the diagnosis? _____

_____

_____

_____

Are there any tests to do? No ☐ Yes ☐          Any procedures to do? No ☐ Yes ☐

What test/procedure & where?_____

_____

_____

_____

Was a prescription given? No ☐   Yes ☐

What is the medicine and dosage?_____

Are there side effects to this medicine? _____

If no medicine was needed, what should I do? _____

What should I do if symptoms return? _____

Where could I get more information? _____

Notes: BP _____ Pulse _____Weight _____Temperature_____ $O_2$ _____

_____

_____

_____

Is there going to be a follow up appointment? No ☐   Yes ☐ When? _____

Actions for me to take: _____

| REMEMBER TO CALL TO CANCEL OR RESCHEDULE YOUR APPOINTMENT IF YOU CAN'T MAKE IT |
| --- |

# DOCTOR'S/PROVIDER'S VISIT NOTES

Day/Date of visit_____Doctor to see _____

Location/Address _____Phone # _____

Directions

_____

_____

Pre-visit instructions?

_____

_____

_____

## BEFORE THE VISIT

Reason for today's visit?

_____

_____

_____

How long has this been going on?

_____

_____

_____

What makes it better or worse?

_____

_____

_____

What have you tried so far?

_____

_____

_____

## NOTES FROM THE VISIT

What is the diagnosis? _____

_____

_____

_____

Are there any tests to do? No ☐ Yes ☐         Any procedures to do? No ☐ Yes ☐

What test/procedure & where?_____

_____

_____

_____

Was a prescription given? No ☐   Yes ☐

What is the medicine and dosage?_____

Are there side effects to this medicine? _____

If no medicine was needed, what should I do? _____

What should I do if symptoms return? _____

Where could I get more information? _____

Notes: BP _____ Pulse _____Weight _____Temperature_____ O$_2$ ____

_____

_____

_____

Is there going to be a follow up appointment? No ☐   Yes ☐ When? _____

Actions for me to take: _____

REMEMBER TO CALL TO CANCEL OR RESCHEDULE YOUR APPOINTMENT IF YOU CAN'T MAKE IT

# DOCTOR'S/PROVIDER'S VISIT NOTES

Day/Date of visit_____Doctor to see _____

Location/Address _____Phone # _____

Directions

_____

_____

Pre-visit instructions?

_____

_____

_____

## BEFORE THE VISIT

Reason for today's visit?

_____

_____

_____

How long has this been going on?

_____

_____

_____

What makes it better or worse?

_____

_____

_____

What have you tried so far?

_____

_____

_____

## NOTES FROM THE VISIT

What is the diagnosis? _____

_____

_____

_____

Are there any tests to do? No ☐ Yes ☐    Any procedures to do? No ☐ Yes ☐

What test/procedure & where?_____

_____

_____

_____

Was a prescription given? No ☐　Yes ☐

What is the medicine and dosage?_____

Are there side effects to this medicine? _____

If no medicine was needed, what should I do? _____

What should I do if symptoms return? _____

Where could I get more information? _____

Notes: BP _____ Pulse _____Weight _____Temperature_____ O$_2$ _____

_____

_____

_____

Is there going to be a follow up appointment? No ☐　Yes ☐ When? _____

Actions for me to take: _____

| REMEMBER TO CALL TO CANCEL OR RESCHEDULE YOUR APPOINTMENT IF YOU CAN'T MAKE IT |
| --- |

# DOCTOR'S/PROVIDER'S VISIT NOTES

Day/Date of visit_____Doctor to see _____

Location/Address _____Phone # _____

Directions

_____

_____

Pre-visit instructions?

_____

_____

_____

## BEFORE THE VISIT

Reason for today's visit?

_____

_____

_____

How long has this been going on?

_____

_____

_____

What makes it better or worse?

_____

_____

_____

What have you tried so far?

_____

_____

_____

## NOTES FROM THE VISIT

What is the diagnosis? _____

_____

_____

_____

Are there any tests to do? No ☐ Yes ☐        Any procedures to do? No ☐ Yes ☐

What test/procedure & where?_____

_____

_____

_____

Was a prescription given? No ☐   Yes ☐

What is the medicine and dosage?_____

Are there side effects to this medicine? _____

If no medicine was needed, what should I do? _____

What should I do if symptoms return? _____

Where could I get more information? _____

Notes: BP _____ Pulse _____Weight _____Temperature_____ O$_2$ _____

_____

_____

_____

Is there going to be a follow up appointment? No ☐   Yes ☐ When? _____

Actions for me to take: _____

**REMEMBER TO CALL TO CANCEL OR RESCHEDULE YOUR APPOINTMENT IF YOU CAN'T MAKE IT**

# DOCTOR'S/PROVIDER'S VISIT NOTES

Day/Date of visit_____ Doctor to see _____

Location/Address _____Phone # _____

Directions

_____

_____

Pre-visit instructions?

_____

_____

_____

## BEFORE THE VISIT

Reason for today's visit?

_____

_____

_____

How long has this been going on?

_____

_____

_____

What makes it better or worse?

_____

_____

_____

What have you tried so far?

_____

_____

_____

## NOTES FROM THE VISIT

What is the diagnosis? _____

_____

_____

_____

Are there any tests to do? No ☐ Yes ☐     Any procedures to do? No ☐ Yes ☐

What test/procedure & where?_____

_____

_____

_____

Was a prescription given? No ☐   Yes ☐

What is the medicine and dosage?_____

Are there side effects to this medicine? _____

If no medicine was needed, what should I do? _____

What should I do if symptoms return? _____

Where could I get more information? _____

Notes: BP _____ Pulse _____ Weight _____ Temperature_____ $O_2$ ____

_____

_____

_____

Is there going to be a follow up appointment? No ☐   Yes ☐ When? _____

Actions for me to take: _____

**REMEMBER TO CALL TO CANCEL OR RESCHEDULE YOUR APPOINTMENT IF YOU CAN'T MAKE IT**

# DOCTOR'S/PROVIDER'S VISIT NOTES

Day/Date of visit_____Doctor to see _____

Location/Address _____Phone # _____

Directions

_____

_____

Pre-visit instructions?

_____

_____

_____

## BEFORE THE VISIT

Reason for today's visit?

_____

_____

_____

How long has this been going on?

_____

_____

_____

What makes it better or worse?

_____

_____

_____

What have you tried so far?

_____

_____

_____

_____

## NOTES FROM THE VISIT

What is the diagnosis? _____

_____

_____

_____

Are there any tests to do? No ☐ Yes ☐    Any procedures to do? No ☐ Yes ☐

What test/procedure & where?_____

_____

_____

_____

Was a prescription given? No ☐   Yes ☐

What is the medicine and dosage?_____

Are there side effects to this medicine? _____

If no medicine was needed, what should I do? _____

What should I do if symptoms return? _____

Where could I get more information? _____

Notes: BP _____ Pulse _____Weight _____Temperature_____ O$_2$____

_____

_____

_____

Is there going to be a follow up appointment? No ☐   Yes ☐ When? _____

Actions for me to take: _____

| REMEMBER TO CALL TO CANCEL OR RESCHEDULE YOUR APPOINTMENT IF YOU CAN'T MAKE IT |
| --- |

# DOCTOR'S/PROVIDER'S VISIT NOTES

Day/Date of visit_____Doctor to see _____

Location/Address _____Phone # _____

Directions

_____

_____

Pre-visit instructions?

_____

_____

_____

## BEFORE THE VISIT

Reason for today's visit?

_____

_____

_____

How long has this been going on?

_____

_____

_____

What makes it better or worse?

_____

_____

_____

What have you tried so far?

_____

_____

_____

## NOTES FROM THE VISIT

What is the diagnosis? _____

_____

_____

_____

Are there any tests to do? No ☐ Yes ☐     Any procedures to do? No ☐ Yes ☐

What test/procedure & where?_____

_____

_____

_____

Was a prescription given? No ☐  Yes ☐

What is the medicine and dosage?_____

Are there side effects to this medicine? _____

If no medicine was needed, what should I do? _____

What should I do if symptoms return? _____

Where could I get more information? _____

Notes: BP _____ Pulse _____Weight _____Temperature_____ O$_2$ ____

_____

_____

_____

Is there going to be a follow up appointment? No ☐  Yes ☐ When? _____

Actions for me to take: _____

**REMEMBER TO CALL TO CANCEL OR RESCHEDULE YOUR APPOINTMENT IF YOU CAN'T MAKE IT**

# DOCTOR'S/PROVIDER'S VISIT NOTES

Day/Date of visit_____Doctor to see _____

Location/Address _____Phone # _____

Directions

_____

_____

Pre-visit instructions?

_____

_____

_____

## BEFORE THE VISIT

Reason for today's visit?

_____

_____

_____

How long has this been going on?

_____

_____

_____

What makes it better or worse?

_____

_____

_____

What have you tried so far?

_____

_____

_____

## NOTES FROM THE VISIT

What is the diagnosis? _____

_____

_____

_____

Are there any tests to do? No ☐ Yes ☐        Any procedures to do? No ☐ Yes ☐

What test/procedure & where?_____

_____

_____

_____

Was a prescription given? No ☐   Yes ☐

What is the medicine and dosage?_____

Are there side effects to this medicine? _____

If no medicine was needed, what should I do? _____

What should I do if symptoms return? _____

Where could I get more information? _____

Notes: BP _____ Pulse _____Weight _____Temperature_____ O$_2$ ____

_____

_____

_____

Is there going to be a follow up appointment? No ☐   Yes ☐ When? _____

Actions for me to take: _____

| REMEMBER TO CALL TO CANCEL OR RESCHEDULE YOUR APPOINTMENT IF YOU CAN'T MAKE IT |

# DOCTOR'S/PROVIDER'S VISIT NOTES

Day/Date of visit_____Doctor to see _____

Location/Address _____Phone # _____

Directions

_____

_____

Pre-visit instructions?

_____

_____

_____

## BEFORE THE VISIT

Reason for today's visit?

_____

_____

_____

How long has this been going on?

_____

_____

_____

What makes it better or worse?

_____

_____

_____

What have you tried so far?

_____

_____

_____

## NOTES FROM THE VISIT

What is the diagnosis? _____

_____

_____

_____

Are there any tests to do? No ☐ Yes ☐     Any procedures to do? No ☐ Yes ☐

What test/procedure & where?_____

_____

_____

_____

Was a prescription given? No ☐   Yes ☐

What is the medicine and dosage?_____

Are there side effects to this medicine? _____

If no medicine was needed, what should I do? _____

What should I do if symptoms return? _____

Where could I get more information? _____

Notes: BP _____ Pulse _____ Weight _____ Temperature_____ O$_2$____

_____

_____

_____

Is there going to be a follow up appointment? No ☐   Yes ☐ When? _____

Actions for me to take: _____

**REMEMBER TO CALL TO CANCEL OR RESCHEDULE YOUR APPOINTMENT IF YOU CAN'T MAKE IT**

# DOCTOR'S/PROVIDER'S VISIT NOTES

Day/Date of visit_____Doctor to see _____

Location/Address _____Phone # _____

Directions

_____

_____

Pre-visit instructions?

_____

_____

_____

## BEFORE THE VISIT

Reason for today's visit?

_____

_____

_____

How long has this been going on?

_____

_____

_____

What makes it better or worse?

_____

_____

_____

What have you tried so far?

_____

_____

_____

What is the diagnosis? _____

_____

_____

_____

Are there any tests to do? No ☐ Yes ☐     Any procedures to do? No ☐ Yes ☐

What test/procedure & where?_____

_____

_____

_____

Was a prescription given? No ☐   Yes ☐

What is the medicine and dosage?_____

Are there side effects to this medicine? _____

If no medicine was needed, what should I do? _____

What should I do if symptoms return? _____

Where could I get more information? _____

Notes: BP _____ Pulse _____ Weight _____ Temperature _____ O$_2$ ____

_____

_____

_____

Is there going to be a follow up appointment? No ☐   Yes ☐ When? _____

Actions for me to take: _____

**REMEMBER TO CALL TO CANCEL OR RESCHEDULE YOUR APPOINTMENT IF YOU CAN'T MAKE IT**

# DOCTOR'S/PROVIDER'S VISIT NOTES

Day/Date of visit_____ Doctor to see _____

Location/Address _____ Phone # _____

Directions

_____

_____

Pre-visit instructions?

_____

_____

_____

## BEFORE THE VISIT

Reason for today's visit?

_____

_____

_____

How long has this been going on?

_____

_____

_____

What makes it better or worse?

_____

_____

_____

What have you tried so far?

_____

_____

_____

## NOTES FROM THE VISIT

What is the diagnosis? _____

_____

_____

_____

Are there any tests to do? No ☐ Yes ☐       Any procedures to do? No ☐ Yes ☐

What test/procedure & where?_____

_____

_____

_____

Was a prescription given? No ☐   Yes ☐

What is the medicine and dosage?_____

Are there side effects to this medicine? _____

If no medicine was needed, what should I do? _____

What should I do if symptoms return? _____

Where could I get more information? _____

Notes: BP _____ Pulse _____Weight _____Temperature_____ O$_2$____

_____

_____

_____

Is there going to be a follow up appointment? No ☐   Yes ☐ When? _____

Actions for me to take: _____

REMEMBER TO CALL TO CANCEL OR RESCHEDULE YOUR APPOINTMENT IF YOU CAN'T MAKE IT

# DOCTOR'S/PROVIDER'S VISIT NOTES

Day/Date of visit_____Doctor to see _____

Location/Address _____Phone # _____

Directions

_____

_____

Pre-visit instructions?

_____

_____

_____

## BEFORE THE VISIT

Reason for today's visit?

_____

_____

_____

How long has this been going on?

_____

_____

_____

What makes it better or worse?

_____

_____

_____

What have you tried so far?

_____

_____

_____

What is the diagnosis? _____

_____

_____

_____

Are there any tests to do? No ☐ Yes ☐    Any procedures to do? No ☐ Yes ☐

What test/procedure & where?_____

_____

_____

_____

Was a prescription given? No ☐   Yes ☐

What is the medicine and dosage?_____

Are there side effects to this medicine? _____

If no medicine was needed, what should I do? _____

What should I do if symptoms return? _____

Where could I get more information? _____

Notes: BP _____ Pulse _____Weight _____Temperature_____ O$_2$ _____

_____

_____

_____

Is there going to be a follow up appointment? No ☐   Yes ☐ When? _____

Actions for me to take: _____

**REMEMBER TO CALL TO CANCEL OR RESCHEDULE YOUR APPOINTMENT IF YOU CAN'T MAKE IT**

# EQUIPMENT LIST

Description of item_____Date received_____

Manufacturer_____Model #_____Serial #_____Size_____

Supplier/Provider_____

Contact Person First and Last Name_____

Phone # (_____)_____Fax # (_____)_____

Email Address_____

Prescribed by_____Phone (_____)_____

Reason prescribed

_____

_____

Description of item_____Date received_____

Manufacturer_____Model #_____Serial #_____Size_____

Supplier/Provider_____

Contact Person First and Last Name_____

Phone # (_____)_____Fax # (_____)_____

Email Address_____

Prescribed by_____Phone (_____)_____

Reason prescribed

_____

_____

# EQUIPMENT LIST

Description of item_____Date received_____

Manufacturer_____Model #_____Serial #_____Size_____

Supplier/Provider_____

Contact Person First and Last Name_____

Phone # (_____)_____Fax # (_____)_____

Email Address_____

Prescribed by_____Phone ( _____ )_____

Reason prescribed

_____
_____

Description of item_____Date received_____

Manufacturer_____Model #_____Serial #_____Size_____

Supplier/Provider_____

Contact Person First and Last Name_____

Phone # (_____)_____Fax # (_____)_____

Email Address_____

Prescribed by_____Phone ( _____ )_____

Reason prescribed

_____
_____

# EQUIPMENT LIST

Description of item_____Date received_____

Manufacturer_____Model #_____Serial #_____Size_____

Supplier/Provider_____

Contact Person First and Last Name_____

Phone # (_____)_____Fax # (_____)_____

Email Address_____

Prescribed by_____Phone (_____)_____

Reason prescribed

_____
_____

Description of item_____Date received_____

Manufacturer_____Model #_____Serial #_____Size_____

Supplier/Provider_____

Contact Person First and Last Name_____

Phone # (_____)_____Fax # (_____)_____

Email Address_____

Prescribed by_____Phone (_____)_____

Reason prescribed

_____
_____

# EQUIPMENT LIST

Description of item_____Date received_____

Manufacturer_____Model #_____Serial #_____Size_____

Supplier/Provider_____

Contact Person First and Last Name_____

Phone # (_____)_____Fax # (_____)_____

Email Address_____

Prescribed by_____Phone (_____)_____

Reason prescribed

_____
_____

Description of item_____Date received_____

Manufacturer_____Model #_____Serial #_____Size_____

Supplier/Provider_____

Contact Person First and Last Name_____

Phone # (_____)_____Fax # (_____)_____

Email Address_____

Prescribed by_____Phone (_____)_____

Reason prescribed

_____
_____

# SUPPLIES LIST

Use this page to track the status of your medical supplies.

| Item # | Product Description | Quantity & Date Ordered |
|---|---|---|
| **Quantity & Date Received** | **Quantity on Backorder** | **Comments** |

| Item # | Product Description | Quantity & Date Ordered |
|---|---|---|
| **Quantity & Date Received** | **Quantity on Backorder** | **Comments** |

| Item # | Product Description | Quantity & Date Ordered |
|---|---|---|
| **Quantity & Date Received** | **Quantity on Backorder** | **Comments** |

| Item # | Product Description | Quantity & Date Ordered |
|---|---|---|
| **Quantity & Date Received** | **Quantity on Backorder** | **Comments** |

# SUPPLIES LIST

Use this page to track the status of your medical supplies.

| Item # | Product Description | Quantity & Date Ordered |
|---|---|---|
| Quantity & Date Received | Quantity on Backorder | Comments |

| Item # | Product Description | Quantity & Date Ordered |
|---|---|---|
| Quantity & Date Received | Quantity on Backorder | Comments |

| Item # | Product Description | Quantity & Date Ordered |
|---|---|---|
| Quantity & Date Received | Quantity on Backorder | Comments |

| Item # | Product Description | Quantity & Date Ordered |
|---|---|---|
| Quantity & Date Received | Quantity on Backorder | Comments |

# SUPPLIES LIST

Use this page to track the status of your medical supplies.

| Item # | Product Description | Quantity & Date Ordered |
|---|---|---|
| Quantity & Date Received | Quantity on Backorder | Comments |

| Item # | Product Description | Quantity & Date Ordered |
|---|---|---|
| Quantity & Date Received | Quantity on Backorder | Comments |

| Item # | Product Description | Quantity & Date Ordered |
|---|---|---|
| Quantity & Date Received | Quantity on Backorder | Comments |

| Item # | Product Description | Quantity & Date Ordered |
|---|---|---|
| Quantity & Date Received | Quantity on Backorder | Comments |

# SUPPLIES LIST

Use this page to track the status of your medical supplies.

| Item # | Product Description | Quantity & Date Ordered |
|---|---|---|
| Quantity & Date Received | Quantity on Backorder | Comments |

| Item # | Product Description | Quantity & Date Ordered |
|---|---|---|
| Quantity & Date Received | Quantity on Backorder | Comments |

| Item # | Product Description | Quantity & Date Ordered |
|---|---|---|
| Quantity & Date Received | Quantity on Backorder | Comments |

| Item # | Product Description | Quantity & Date Ordered |
|---|---|---|
| Quantity & Date Received | Quantity on Backorder | Comments |

# Section 4
# Health History

❖ **My Health History**
❖ **My Family Health History**
❖ **Surgeries & Procedures**
❖ **Emergency Calls**
❖ **Hospital Admission Tracking**
**(*Other than surgery*)**
❖ **My Test Results Log (*include records
of blood or urine tests, X-rays, etc.*)**
❖ **Medical Records from Doctors**

# MY FAMILY HEALTH HISTORY

My Name _____

My Nickname _____

SSN_____

Date of Birth _____

Have any family members had genetic testing/counseling? Yes ☐ No ☐
Unsure ☐

**Past Medical History** – Please check all that apply to you:

| | | |
|---|---|---|
| ☐ Arthritis | ☐ Epilepsy / seizures | ☐ Migraine |
| ☐ Cancer | ☐ Gastrointestinal issues | ☐ Psychiatric disorder/disease |
| ☐ Constipation | ☐ Heart problems | ☐ Stroke |
| ☐ Depression | ☐ Heart surgery | ☐ Thyroid |
| ☐ Diabetes | ☐ High blood pressure | ☐ None |

Injuries: list any injuries you have had_____

_____

Allergies: list any allergies that you have:

_____

_____

Do you drink alcohol?  Yes ☐   No ☐ If yes, how much / week? _____

Do you smoke?  Yes ☐   No ☐ If yes, what do you smoke and how many / day?

_____

Do you consume caffeine?  Yes ☐   No ☐ If yes, what form (i.e. coffee) and how

many cups / day? _____

Do you use recreational drugs?  Yes ☐   No ☐ If yes, what type and frequency?

_____

Are you on a special diet?  Yes ☐   No ☐ If yes, please describe

_____

**Family Medical History** – To your knowledge, have any of your blood relatives have / had the following:

| | | |
|---|---|---|
| ☐ Arthritis | ☐ Headaches | ☐ Psychiatric disorder/disease, Type |
| ☐ Asthma | ☐ Heart problems | |
| ☐ Brain Tumor | ☐ Heart surgery | _____ |
| ☐ Cancer, Type | ☐ High blood pressure | ☐ Stroke |
| _____ | ☐ Kidney disease | ☐ Thyroid |
| ☐ Constipation | ☐ Lung disease | ☐ Ulcers |
| ☐ Depression | ☐ Migraine | ☐ Urinary tract infections |
| ☐ Diabetes | ☐ Multiple Sclerosis | |
| ☐ Epilepsy / seizures | ☐ Muscle disease | ☐ None |
| ☐ Gastrointestinal issues | | |

**Family Medical History** – To your knowledge, have you or any of your blood relatives (have) had the following: **General Health**

☐ Good general health
☐ Recent weight change
☐ Loss of appetite
☐ Fatigue
☐ Fever / chills

**Allergy**
☐ Drug allergies
☐ Food allergies
☐ Hay fever
☐ Other: _____
☐ None

**Ears, Nose, Mouth, Throat**
☐ Difficulty swallowing
☐ Earaches
☐ Loss of hearing/deaf
☐ Loss of taste
☐ Painful chewing

**Eyes**
☐ Blind spots
☐ Blurred vision
☐ Double vision
☐ Glaucoma
☐ Injury
☐ Pain
☐ Other
_____
☐ None

**Muscles / Joints / Bones**
☐ Back pain
☐ Difficulty walking
☐ Joint pain
☐ Joint stiffness or swelling
☐ Muscle pain or tenderness
☐ Neck pain
☐ None

Are you?
☐ Right handed

**Gastrointestinal**
☐ Blood in stools
☐ Increasing constipation
☐ Nausea
☐ Painful bowel movements
☐ Persistent diarrhea
☐ Stomach or abdominal pain
☐ Ulcer
☐ Vomiting
☐ Other
_____
☐ None

- ☐ Ringing in ears
- ☐ Sinus infection
- ☐ Sores in mouth
- ☐ None

**Genitourinary**
- ☐ Blood in urine
- ☐ Female: irregular periods
- ☐ Female: # pregnancies
- ☐ _____
- ☐ Female # miscarriages

  _____
- ☐ Female: vaginal discharge
- ☐ Kidney stones
- ☐ Male: Prostate disease
- ☐ Male: testicle pain
- ☐ Male: Erectile dysfunction
- ☐ Painful or burning urination
- ☐ Sexual difficulty
- ☐ Sexually transmitted disease
- ☐ Urgency with urination
- ☐ Urine retention/incontinence
- ☐ Other _____
- ☐ None

**Heart and Lungs**
- ☐ Pain in chest
- ☐ High blood pressure
- ☐ High cholesterol
- ☐ Irregular heart beat
- ☐ Other _____
- ☐ None

- ☐ Left handed
- ☐ Both

**Neurological**
- ☐ Balance trouble
- ☐ Black outs / loss of consciousness
- ☐ Difficulty speaking
- ☐ Difficulty walking
- ☐ Facial drooping
- ☐ Headaches
- ☐ Injury to the brain or spine
- ☐ Light-headed or dizziness
- ☐ Memory loss
- ☐ Mental confusion
- ☐ Migraines
- ☐ Mini stroke
- ☐ Neuropathy
- ☐ Numbness or tingling
- ☐ Paralysis
- ☐ Stroke
- ☐ Tremors
- ☐ Weakness
- ☐ Other _____
- ☐ None

Are you?
- ☐ Right handed
- ☐ Left handed
- ☐ Both

**Psychiatric**
- ☐ Depression
- ☐ Anxiety
- ☐ Eating disorder
- ☐ Other:

  _____
- ☐ None

**Pulmonary**
- ☐ Asthma
- ☐ Blood in cough
- ☐ Cancer
- ☐ Chronic or frequent cough
- ☐ Emphysema
- ☐ Pneumonia
- ☐ Shortness of breath
- ☐ Other:

  _____
- ☐ None

**Skin**
- ☐ Rash or itching
- ☐ Sun sensitivity
- ☐ Hair loss
- ☐ Color changes
- ☐ Other:

  _____
- ☐ None

**Sleep**
- ☐ Snoring
- ☐ Sleep waling
- ☐ Night mares

Do you sleep well?
Yes ☐   No ☐

| | | Do you feel rested when you wake? Yes ☐ No ☐ |
| --- | --- | --- |
| | | Do you fall asleep during the day? Yes ☐ No ☐ |

# Notes and Reflections

# SURGERIES & PROCEDURES

Use this log to track surgeries and medical procedures.

| Description of Surgery or Procedure | Surgeon or Provider/Hospital | Date(s) From – To |
|---|---|---|
| | | |
| | | |
| | | |
| | | |
| | | |
| | | |
| | | |
| | | |

# SURGERIES & PROCEDURES

Use this log to track surgeries and medical procedures.

| Description of Surgery or Procedure | Surgeon or Provider/Hospital | Date(s) From – To |
|---|---|---|
| | | |
| | | |
| | | |
| | | |
| | | |
| | | |
| | | |
| | | |

# Emergency Calls

Use this log to track calls for emergencies.

| Reason For Call | Who Responded | Date(s) From – To |
|---|---|---|
|  |  |  |
|  |  |  |
|  |  |  |
|  |  |  |
|  |  |  |
|  |  |  |
|  |  |  |
|  |  |  |

# Emergency Calls

Use this log to track calls for emergencies.

| Reason For Call | Who Responded | Date(s) From – To |
|---|---|---|
| | | |
| | | |
| | | |
| | | |
| | | |
| | | |
| | | |
| | | |

# HOSPITAL ADMISSIONS TRACKING

Use this log to track hospital admissions for reasons other than surgery

| Reason For Admission | Hospital | Date(s) From – To |
|---|---|---|
| | | |
| | | |
| | | |
| | | |
| | | |
| | | |
| | | |
| | | |

# HOSPITAL ADMISSIONS TRACKING

Use this log to track hospital admissions for reasons other than surgery

| Reason For Admission | Hospital | Date(s) From – To |
|---|---|---|
|  |  |  |
|  |  |  |
|  |  |  |
|  |  |  |
|  |  |  |
|  |  |  |
|  |  |  |
|  |  |  |

# MY TEST RESULTS LOG

Use this form to keep a record of all of your tests in one convenient location

Type of test: **Blood** ☐ **X-ray** ☐ **CT** ☐ **MRI** ☐ **EEG** ☐

**Other** ☐ _____ **Date of test:** _____

Description of test _____

Doctor who ordered test _____ Phone # (____) _____

Location where test was performed _____ Phone # (____) _____

Results _____

Comments _____

_____

---

Type of test: **Blood** ☐ **X-ray** ☐ **CT** ☐ **MRI** ☐ **EEG** ☐

**Other** ☐ _____ **Date of test:** _____

Description of test _____

Doctor who ordered test _____ Phone # (____) _____

Location where test was performed _____ Phone # (____) _____

Results _____

Comments _____

_____

# MY TEST RESULTS LOG

Use this form to keep a record of all of your tests in one convenient location

Type of test: **Blood** ☐ **X-ray** ☐ **CT** ☐ **MRI** ☐ **EEG** ☐

**Other** ☐ _____ **Date of test:** _____

Description of test _____

Doctor who ordered test _____ Phone # (____) _____

Location where test was performed _____ Phone # (____) _____

Results _____

Comments _____
_____

---

Type of test: **Blood** ☐ **X-ray** ☐ **CT** ☐ **MRI** ☐ **EEG** ☐

**Other** ☐ _____ **Date of test:** _____

Description of test _____

Doctor who ordered test _____ Phone # (____) _____

Location where test was performed _____ Phone # (____) _____

Results _____

Comments _____
_____

# MY TEST RESULTS LOG

Use this form to keep a record of all of your tests in one convenient location

Type of test: **Blood** ☐  **X-ray** ☐  **CT** ☐  **MRI** ☐  **EEG** ☐

**Other** ☐ _____  **Date of test:** _____

Description of test _____

Doctor who ordered test _____ Phone # (____) _____

Location where test was performed _____ Phone # (____) _____

Results _____

Comments _____
_____

---

Type of test: **Blood** ☐  **X-ray** ☐  **CT** ☐  **MRI** ☐  **EEG** ☐

**Other** ☐ _____  **Date of test:** _____

Description of test _____

Doctor who ordered test _____ Phone # (____) _____

Location where test was performed _____ Phone # (____) _____

Results _____

Comments _____
_____

# MY TEST RESULTS LOG

Use this form to keep a record of all of your tests in one convenient location

Type of test: **Blood** ☐  **X-ray** ☐ **CT** ☐ **MRI** ☐ **EEG** ☐

**Other** ☐ _____  **Date of test:** _____

Description of test _____

Doctor who ordered test _____ Phone # (_____) _____

Location where test was performed _____ Phone # (_____) _____

Results _____

Comments _____

_____

---

Type of test: **Blood** ☐  **X-ray** ☐ **CT** ☐ **MRI** ☐ **EEG** ☐

**Other** ☐ _____  **Date of test:** _____

Description of test _____

Doctor who ordered test _____ Phone # (_____) _____

Location where test was performed _____ Phone # (_____) _____

Results _____

Comments _____

_____

# Section 5
# Medication Management


❖ **Medication Management Logs**
❖ **Diet & Nutrition Notes**

# MEDICATION LIST

My name is _____  My birthday is _____ / ____ / _____

Pharmacy Name _____Phone_____

Pharmacy Address _____

Primary Care Physician_____

**Copy form as needed**

| DRUG NAME | DOSAGE | FREQUENCY | INDICATION FOR TAKING |
|---|---|---|---|
| *Example: Telmisartan* | *80 mg tablet* | *Once a day* | *High Blood Pressure* |
| | | | |
| | | | |
| | | | |
| | | | |
| | | | |
| | | | |
| | | | |
| | | | |
| | | | |
| | | | |
| | | | |
| | | | |
| | | | |
| | | | |
| | | | |
| | | | |
| | | | |

Allergies _____

Patient Signature _____ Date _____

# MEDICATION LIST

My name is _____ My birthday is _____ / ___ / _____
Pharmacy Name _____Phone_____
Pharmacy Address _____
Primary Care Physician_____

**Copy form as needed**

| DRUG NAME | DOSAGE | FREQUENCY | INDICATION FOR TAKING |
|---|---|---|---|
| *Example: Telmisartan* | *80 mg tablet* | *Once a day* | *High Blood Pressure* |
| | | | |
| | | | |
| | | | |
| | | | |
| | | | |
| | | | |
| | | | |
| | | | |
| | | | |
| | | | |
| | | | |
| | | | |
| | | | |
| | | | |
| | | | |
| | | | |
| | | | |

Allergies _____

Patient Signature _____ Date _____

# MEDICATION LIST

My name is _____ My birthday is _____/____/_____

Pharmacy Name _____Phone_____

Pharmacy Address _____

Primary Care Physician_____

**Copy form as needed**

| DRUG NAME | DOSAGE | FREQUENCY | INDICATION FOR TAKING |
|---|---|---|---|
| *Example: Telmisartan* | *80 mg tablet* | *Once a day* | *High Blood Pressure* |
| | | | |
| | | | |
| | | | |
| | | | |
| | | | |
| | | | |
| | | | |
| | | | |
| | | | |
| | | | |
| | | | |
| | | | |
| | | | |
| | | | |
| | | | |
| | | | |
| | | | |

Allergies _____

Patient Signature _____ Date _____

# MEDICATION MANAGEMENT FORM

My name is _____ My birthday is _____ / ___ / _____

Pharmacy Name _____

Pharmacy Address _____

Pharmacy Phone _____

| Name of Medicine (brand/generic) | Dosage (mg, units, puffs, drops) | How often taken? | Reason for taking/treatment of |
|---|---|---|---|
| Start Date | End Date | Prescribed by | Additional notes including side effects/Danger signs |
| | | | |
| Name of Medicine (brand/generic) | Dosage (mg, units, puffs, drops) | How often taken? | Reason for taking/treatment of |
| Start Date | End Date | Prescribed by | Additional notes including side effects/Danger signs |
| | | | |
| Name of Medicine (brand/generic) | Dosage (mg, units, puffs, drops) | How often taken? | Reason for taking/treatment of |
| Start Date | End Date | Prescribed by | Additional notes including side effects/Danger signs |
| | | | |

| Name of Medicine (brand/generic) | Dosage (mg, units, puffs, drops) | How often taken? | Reason for taking/treatment of |
|---|---|---|---|
| Start Date | End Date | Prescribed by | Additional notes including side effects/Danger signs |

| Name of Medicine (brand/generic) | Dosage (mg, units, puffs, drops) | How often taken? | Reason for taking/treatment of |
|---|---|---|---|
| Start Date | End Date | Prescribed by | Additional notes including side effects/Danger signs |

| Name of Medicine (brand/generic) | Dosage (mg, units, puffs, drops) | How often taken? | Reason for taking/treatment of |
|---|---|---|---|
| Start Date | End Date | Prescribed by | Additional notes including side effects/Danger signs |

| Name of Medicine (brand/generic) | Dosage (mg, units, puffs, drops) | How often taken? | Reason for taking/treatment of |
|---|---|---|---|
| Start Date | End Date | Prescribed by | Additional notes including side effects/Danger signs |

| Name of Medicine (brand/generic) | Dosage (mg, units, puffs, drops) | How often taken? | Reason for taking/treatment of |
|---|---|---|---|
| Start Date | End Date | Prescribed by | Additional notes including side effects/Danger signs |

| Name of Medicine (brand/generic) | Dosage (mg, units, puffs, drops) | How often taken? | Reason for taking/treatment of |
|---|---|---|---|
| Start Date | End Date | Prescribed by | Additional notes including side effects/Danger signs |

| Name of Medicine (brand/generic) | Dosage (mg, units, puffs, drops) | How often taken? | Reason for taking/treatment of |
|---|---|---|---|
| Start Date | End Date | Prescribed by | Additional notes including side effects/Danger signs |

| Name of Medicine (brand/generic) | Dosage (mg, units, puffs, drops) | How often taken? | Reason for taking/treatment of |
|---|---|---|---|
| Start Date | End Date | Prescribed by | Additional notes including side effects/Danger signs |

| Name of Medicine (brand/generic) | Dosage (mg, units, puffs, drops) | How often taken? | Reason for taking/treatment of |
|---|---|---|---|
| Start Date | End Date | Prescribed by | Additional notes including side effects/Danger signs |

| Name of Medicine (brand/generic) | Dosage (mg, units, puffs, drops) | How often taken? | Reason for taking/treatment of |
|---|---|---|---|
| Start Date | End Date | Prescribed by | Additional notes including side effects/Danger signs |

| Name of Medicine (brand/generic) | Dosage (mg, units, puffs, drops) | How often taken? | Reason for taking/treatment of |
|---|---|---|---|
| Start Date | End Date | Prescribed by | Additional notes including side effects/Danger signs |

| Name of Medicine (brand/generic) | Dosage (mg, units, puffs, drops) | How often taken? | Reason for taking/treatment of |
|---|---|---|---|
| Start Date | End Date | Prescribed by | Additional notes including side effects/Danger signs |

| Name of Medicine (brand/generic) | Dosage (mg, units, puffs, drops) | How often taken? | Reason for taking/treatment of |
|---|---|---|---|
| Start Date | End Date | Prescribed by | Additional notes including side effects/Danger signs |

| Name of Medicine (brand/generic) | Dosage (mg, units, puffs, drops) | How often taken? | Reason for taking/treatment of |
|---|---|---|---|
| Start Date | End Date | Prescribed by | Additional notes including side effects/Danger signs |

| Name of Medicine (brand/generic) | Dosage (mg, units, puffs, drops) | How often taken? | Reason for taking/treatment of |
|---|---|---|---|
| Start Date | End Date | Prescribed by | Additional notes including side effects/Danger signs |

| Name of Medicine (brand/generic) | Dosage (mg, units, puffs, drops) | How often taken? | Reason for taking/treatment of |
|---|---|---|---|
| Start Date | End Date | Prescribed by | Additional notes including side effects/Danger signs |

| Name of Medicine (brand/generic) | Dosage (mg, units, puffs, drops) | How often taken? | Reason for taking/treatment of |
|---|---|---|---|
| Start Date | End Date | Prescribed by | Additional notes including side effects/Danger signs |

| Name of Medicine (brand/generic) | Dosage (mg, units, puffs, drops) | How often taken? | Reason for taking/treatment of |
|---|---|---|---|
| Start Date | End Date | Prescribed by | Additional notes including side effects/Danger signs |

| Name of Medicine (brand/generic) | Dosage (mg, units, puffs, drops) | How often taken? | Reason for taking/treatment of |
|---|---|---|---|
| Start Date | End Date | Prescribed by | Additional notes including side effects/Danger signs |

| Name of Medicine (brand/generic) | Dosage (mg, units, puffs, drops) | How often taken? | Reason for taking/treatment of |
|---|---|---|---|
| Start Date | End Date | Prescribed by | Additional notes including side effects/Danger signs |

| Name of Medicine (brand/generic) | Dosage (mg, units, puffs, drops) | How often taken? | Reason for taking/treatment of |
|---|---|---|---|
| Start Date | End Date | Prescribed by | Additional notes including side effects/Danger signs |

| Name of Medicine (brand/generic) | Dosage (mg, units, puffs, drops) | How often taken? | Reason for taking/treatment of |
|---|---|---|---|
| Start Date | End Date | Prescribed by | Additional notes including side effects/Danger signs |

| Name of Medicine (brand/generic) | Dosage (mg, units, puffs, drops) | How often taken? | Reason for taking/treatment of |
|---|---|---|---|
| Start Date | End Date | Prescribed by | Additional notes including side effects/Danger signs |

| Name of Medicine (brand/generic) | Dosage (mg, units, puffs, drops) | How often taken? | Reason for taking/treatment of |
|---|---|---|---|
| Start Date | End Date | Prescribed by | Additional notes including side effects/Danger signs |

| Name of Medicine (brand/generic) | Dosage (mg, units, puffs, drops) | How often taken? | Reason for taking/treatment of |
|---|---|---|---|
| Start Date | End Date | Prescribed by | Additional notes including side effects/Danger signs |

| Name of Medicine (brand/generic) | Dosage (mg, units, puffs, drops) | How often taken? | Reason for taking/treatment of |
|---|---|---|---|
| Start Date | End Date | Prescribed by | Additional notes including side effects/Danger signs |

| Name of Medicine (brand/generic) | Dosage (mg, units, puffs, drops) | How often taken? | Reason for taking/treatment of |
|---|---|---|---|
| Start Date | End Date | Prescribed by | Additional notes including side effects/Danger signs |

| Name of Medicine (brand/generic) | Dosage (mg, units, puffs, drops) | How often taken? | Reason for taking/treatment of |
|---|---|---|---|
| Start Date | End Date | Prescribed by | Additional notes including side effects/Danger signs |

# DIET & NUTRITION NOTES

Use this page to write about your nutritional needs. Describe foods and any nutritional formulas you take, any food allergies or restrictions. Include any special feeding techniques, precautions, or equipment used for feedings. This form will be especially helpful for times if/when someone else helps to provide care for you.

I take my food by: ☐ Mouth  ☐ G-tube  ☐GJ tube  ☐NG  ☐ NJ Size of Tube_____

| Date | Breakfast | Lunch |
|------|-----------|-------|
| Dinner | Snacks | Notes |
| Date | Breakfast | Lunch |
| Dinner | Snacks | Notes |
| Date | Breakfast | Lunch |
| Dinner | Snacks | Notes |

### Food Allergies / Restrictions & Additional Notes

Food _____ Reaction _____

Food _____ Reaction _____

Food _____ Reaction _____

_____

_____

_____

# Notes and Reflections

# Section 6
# Insurance
# Information

❖ **Insurance information**
❖ **Record of Medical Expenses**

# INSURANCE INFORMATION

## PRIMARY INSURANCE POLICY

Insurance Company Name _____Phone # (_____)_____

Insurance Policy Number _____Group  #_____

Co-Pay _____Deducible _____

### Policy Holder's Information

Name _____Date of Birth _____

Employer's Name _____

 Employer's Address _____

City _____ State _____ Zip Code _____

Phone # (_____) _____ Fax # (_____) _____

## SECONDARY INSURANCE POLICY

Insurance Company Name _____Phone # (_____)_____

Insurance Policy Number _____Group  #_____

Co-Pay _____Deducible _____

### Policy Holder's Information

Name _____Date of Birth _____

Employer's Name _____

Employer's Address _____

City _____ State _____ Zip Code _____

Phone # (_____) _____ Fax # (_____) _____

# INSURANCE INFORMATION

## OTHER INSURANCE POLICY

Insurance Company Name _____ Phone # (____) _____

Insurance Policy Number _____ Group # _____

Co-Pay _____ Deducible _____

### Policy Holder's Information

Name _____ Date of Birth _____

Employer's Name _____

Employer's Address _____

City _____ State _____ Zip Code _____

Phone # (____) _____ Fax # (____) _____

## OTHER / DISCOUNT PROGRAM

Company Name _____ Phone # (____) _____

Company Policy Number _____ Group # _____

Co-Pay _____ Deducible _____

### Policy Holder's Information

Name _____ Date of Birth _____

Employer's Name _____

Employer's Address _____

City _____ State _____ Zip Code _____

Phone # (____) _____ Fax # (____) _____

# Notes and Reflections

_____
_____
_____
_____
_____
_____
_____
_____
_____
_____
_____
_____
_____
_____
_____
_____
_____
_____
_____
_____
_____
_____
_____

# RECORD OF MEDICAL EXPENSES

Use this log to track expenses that you have that are not covered by insurance including driving mileage to/from medical appointments. Make sure to save all receipts for tax purposes.

| Date paid | Name of person paid | Address of person paid or provider seen | Amount paid | Description of fee/service or item (i.e. taxi, mileage, parking, etc.) |
|---|---|---|---|---|
| | | | | |
| | | | | |
| | | | | |
| | | | | |
| | | | | |
| | | | | |
| | | | | |

# Notes and Reflections

# Section 7
# Doctor and Business Contacts

## List Contents

❖ **Primary Care Providers Contact Information**
❖ **Specialist Providers Contact Information**
❖ **General Providers Contact Information**
❖ **May include some or all of the following:**

- Exercise/ Recreation Center
- Dental Care Provider
- Home Health Care Provider
- Insurance Case Manager
- Durable Medical Equipment Provider

- Medicaid
- Transportation
- Social Services
- Respite Care

- Therapists
- Elder Care
- Hospice Services
- Clinic Coordinator

❖ **Business Card pages**

# Notes and Reflections

_____
_____
_____
_____
_____
_____
_____
_____
_____
_____
_____
_____
_____
_____
_____
_____
_____
_____
_____
_____
_____
_____

# PRIMARY & SPECIALTY CARE PHYSICIANS

## PRIMARY CARE PHYSICIAN/PROVIDER

**Name of Doctor/Provider**_____

Contact Person First and Last Name _____

Location/Address _____

City_____ State _____ Zip Code _____

Directions _____

Phone # (_____) _____ Fax # (_____)_____

Hours of operation _____

Date care started _____ Date care ended _____

## SPECIALIST/PROVIDER FOR _____

**Name of Doctor/Provider**_____

Contact Person First and Last Name _____

Location/Address _____

City_____ State _____ Zip Code _____

Directions _____

Phone # (_____) _____ Fax # (_____)_____

Hours of operation _____

Date care started _____ Date care ended _____

# PRIMARY & SPECIALTY CARE PHYSICIANS

**SPECIALIST/PROVIDER FOR** _____

**Name of Doctor/Provider** _____

Contact Person First and Last Name _____

Location/Address _____

City_____ State _____ Zip Code _____

Directions _____

_____

Phone # (_____) _____ Fax # (_____)_____

Hours of operation _____

Date care started _____ Date care ended _____

**SPECIALIST/PROVIDER FOR** _____

**Name of Doctor/Provider** _____

Contact Person First and Last Name _____

Location/Address _____

City_____ State _____ Zip Code _____

Directions _____

_____

Phone # (_____) _____ Fax # (_____)_____

Hours of operation _____

Date care started _____ Date care ended _____

# PRIMARY & SPECIALTY CARE PHYSICIANS

**SPECIALIST/PROVIDER FOR** _____

**Name of Doctor/Provider** _____

Contact Person First and Last Name _____

Location/Address _____

City_____ State _____Zip Code _____

Directions _____

Phone # (_____) _____ Fax # (_____)_____

Hours of operation _____

Date care started _____ Date care ended _____

**SPECIALIST/PROVIDER FOR** _____

**Name of Doctor/Provider** _____

Contact Person First and Last Name _____

Location/Address _____

City_____ State _____Zip Code _____

Directions _____

Phone # (_____) _____ Fax # (_____)_____

Hours of operation _____

Date care started _____ Date care ended _____

# PRIMARY & SPECIALTY CARE PHYSICIANS

**SPECIALIST/PROVIDER FOR** _____

**Name of Doctor/Provider**_____

Contact Person First and Last Name _____

Location/Address _____

City_____ State _____ Zip Code _____

Directions _____

Phone # (_____) _____ Fax # (_____)_____

Hours of operation _____

Date care started _____ Date care ended _____

**SPECIALIST/PROVIDER FOR** _____

**Name of Doctor/Provider**_____

Contact Person First and Last Name _____

Location/Address _____

City_____ State _____ Zip Code _____

Directions _____

Phone # (_____) _____ Fax # (_____)_____

Hours of operation _____

Date care started _____ Date care ended _____

# PRIMARY & SPECIALTY CARE PHYSICIANS

**SPECIALIST/PROVIDER FOR** _____

**Name of Doctor/Provider**_____

Contact Person First and Last Name _____

Location/Address _____

City_____ State _____ Zip Code _____

Directions _____

_____

Phone # (_____) _____ Fax # (_____)_____

Hours of operation _____

Date care started _____ Date care ended _____

**SPECIALIST/PROVIDER FOR** _____

**Name of Doctor/Provider**_____

Contact Person First and Last Name _____

Location/Address _____

City_____ State _____ Zip Code _____

Directions _____

_____

Phone # (_____) _____ Fax # (_____)_____

Hours of operation _____

Date care started _____ Date care ended _____

# BUSINESS CARDS
*(TAPE HERE)*

# BUSINESS CARDS
*(TAPE HERE)*

# BUSINESS CARDS
*(TAPE HERE)*

# Section 8
# Miscellaneous
# Documents

*(Insert copies of correspondence including appointment letters, insurance referral authorization letter, etc.)*

# Notes and Reflections

# About the Authors

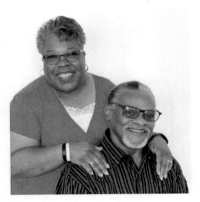

John and Monette Mottenon are a couple committed to each other and their health. Living with chronic illnesses, they needed a way to track their health information. The ***My Health Information Planner*** was created to help them and others maintain accurate records of their health. They are excited to be able to share this and help others improve the quality of their life. John and Monette live in Montgomery, Alabama and have a large blended family that they enjoy.

Made in the USA
Monee, IL
09 October 2022

15186222R00100